The World Health Organization is a specialized agency of the United Nations with primary responsibility for international health matters and public health. Through this organization, which was created in 1948, the health professions of some 190 countries exchange their knowledge and experience with the aim of making possible the attainment by all citizens of the world by the year 2000 of a level of health that will permit them to lead a socially and economically productive life.

By means of direct technical cooperation with its Member States, and by stimulating such cooperation among them, WHO promotes the development of comprehensive health services, the prevention and control of diseases, the improvement of environmental conditions, the development of human resources for health, the coordination and development of biomedical and health services research, and the planning and implementation of health programmes.

These broad fields of endeavour encompass a wide variety of activities, such as developing systems of primary health care that reach the whole population of Member countries; promoting the health of mothers and children; combating malnutrition, controlling malaria and other communicable diseases including tuberculosis and leprosy; coordinating the global strategy for the prevention and control of AIDS; having achieved the eradication of smallpox, promoting mass immunization against a number of other preventable diseases; improving mental health; providing safe water supplies; and training health personnel of all categories.

Progress towards better health throughout the world also demands international cooperation in such matters as establishing international standards for biological substances, pesticides and pharmaceuticals; formulating environmental health criteria; recommending international nonproprietary names for drugs; administering the International Health Regulations; revising the International Statistical Classification of Diseases and Related Health Problems and collecting and disseminating health statistical information.

Reflecting the concerns and priorities of the Organization and its Member States, WHO publications provide authoritative information and guidance aimed at promoting and protecting health and preventing and controlling disease.

Basic analytical toxicology

R.J. Flanagan
Guy's and St Thomas' Hospital NHS Trust
London, England

R.A. Braithwaite
Regional Laboratory for Toxicology
City Hospital NHS Trust
Birmingham, England

S.S. Brown
Formerly Regional Laboratory for Toxicology
City Hospital NHS Trust
Birmingham, England

B. Widdop
Guy's and St Thomas' Hospital NHS Trust
London, England

F.A. de Wolff
Department of Human Toxicology, Academic Medical Centre
University of Amsterdam
Amsterdam, Netherlands

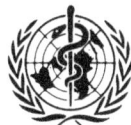

World Health Organization
Geneva
1995

WHO Library Cataloguing in Publication Data

Basic analytical toxicology / R. J. Flanagan. . .[et al.].

  1.Poisoning 2.Poisons — analysis 3.Toxicology — laboratory manuals
  I.Flanagan, R. J.

  ISBN 92 4 154458 9   (NLM Classification: QV 602)

TYPESET IN INDIA
PRINTED IN ENGLAND

92/9443—Macmillan/Clays/TWC—5000

Contents

Preface

For many years, toxicology, the science of poisons and poisoning, was considered to be no more than a branch of forensic science and criminology. Nowadays, it is clear that the study of applied toxicology in its various forms — clinical, occupational, forensic, nutritional, veterinary, and environmental toxicology, ecotoxicology and related areas — is important, if not vital, to the continued development of life on earth. Yet toxicology is rarely taught as a subject in its own right and then mostly at postgraduate level. In consequence, most toxicologists come to the subject under the auspices of another discipline. Clinical toxicology, dealing with the prevention, diagnosis and management of poisoning, is no exception, being often thought of as a branch of emergency medicine and intensive care on the one hand, and of clinical pharmacology on the other.

The provision of services for the management of poisoned patients varies greatly, from specialized treatment units to, more commonly, general emergency medicine. Analytical toxicology services, which provide support for the diagnosis, prognosis and management of poisoning, are also variable and dependent on local arrangements. In developed countries, they may be provided by a specialized laboratory attached to a clinical toxicology unit, by a hospital biochemistry laboratory, an analytical pharmacy unit, a university department of forensic medicine, or a government forensic science laboratory.

In many developing countries, such services are not available on a regular basis, and where they are available, the physician is generally dependent on a national or regional health laboratory established for other purposes and operating only part of the time. There are, however, many simple analytical techniques that do not need sophisticated equipment or expensive reagents, or even a continuous supply of electricity. Such tests could be carried out in the basic laboratories that are available to most hospitals and health facilities, even in developing countries. With training, hospital laboratory staff could use these techniques to provide an analytical toxicology service to the physicians treating poisoned patients.

This manual, which describes simple analytical techniques of this kind, has been prepared on the recommendation of a group of experts, convened by the International Programme on Chemical Safety (IPCS)[a] in February 1987.

The draft text was reviewed by a number of experts, as noted under "Acknowledgements", and the procedures described were tested in the laboratory, as far as possible by technicians from developing countries. The work was coordinated for IPCS by Dr J. Haines. The United Kingdom Department of Health, through its financial support to the IPCS, provided the resources for the editorial group to meet and undertake its work.

The aim of this manual is to help hospital laboratories in developing countries to provide a basic analytical toxicology service using a minimum of special apparatus. It is not intended to replace standard texts, but to provide practical information on the analysis of a number of substances frequently involved in acute poisoning incidents. Common pitfalls and problems are emphasized throughout, and basic health and safety precautions for laboratory workers are also discussed.

Problems encountered when using relatively simple methods in analytical toxicology are usually due to interference (false positives) or poor sensitivity (false negatives). Nevertheless, useful information to help the clinician, and thus the patient, can often be obtained if the tests are applied with due caution using an appropriate sample. While every effort has been made to ensure that the tests described are reliable and accurate, no responsibility can be accepted by UNEP, ILO or WHO for the use made of the tests or of the results obtained.

As in all areas of analytical chemistry, problems in interpretation can arise if a result is used for purposes for which it was not intended. This is especially true if the results of emergency toxicological analyses, particularly if poorly defined (for example, "negative drug screen", "opiates positive"), are used as evidence in legal proceedings many months or even years later. In this context, the importance of consultation between the clinician treating the patient and the analyst in making best use of the analytical facilities available cannot be overemphasized. To assist this dialogue, some information on clinical interpretation has been included.

IPCS and the editorial group would welcome comments on the content and structure of the manual; such comments should be addressed in the first instance to the Director, International Programme on

---

[a] The IPCS is a cooperative programme of the United Nations Environment Programme (UNEP), the International Labour Organisation (ILO) and the World Health Organization (WHO). WHO is the executing agency for the programme, which aims to provide the internationally evaluated scientific data basis for countries to develop their own chemical safety measures and to strengthen national capabilities to prevent and treat harmful effects of chemicals and to manage chemical emergencies.

Chemical Safety, World Health Organization, 1211 Geneva 27, Switzerland. Two areas for further development have already been identified, namely, the requirement for formal training in analytical toxicology, and the need to ensure the supply of essential reference compounds, specialized reagents and laboratory consumables. Comments on either of these problems would also be welcome.

Acknowledgements

Many individuals have contributed to the preparation of this manual by providing support, ideas, details of methods or comments on various drafts. In particular, Professor Bahira Fahim, Cairo, Egypt, Dr I. Sunshine, Palo Alto, CA, USA, and Dr G. Volans, London, England provided initial encouragement. Dr T. J. Meredith, London, England, Dr J. Pronczuk de Garbino, Montevideo, Uruguay, and Professor A. N. P. van Heijst, Utrecht, Netherlands scrutinized the clinical information. Dr A. Akintonwa, Lagos, Nigeria, Dr A. Badawy, Cairo, Egypt, Dr N. Besbelli, Ankara, Turkey, Dr C. Heuck, WHO, Geneva, Switzerland, Professor M. Geldmacher-von Mallinckrodt, Erlangen, Germany, Mr R. Fysh, London, England, Professor R. Merad, Algiers, Algeria, and Mr. J. Ramsey, Mr J. Slaughterr and Dr J. Taylor, London, England kindly commented on various aspects of the final draft. Miss H. Triador, Montevideo, Uruguay, Mrs K. Pumala, Bangkok, Thailand and Mr J. Howard, London, England, undertook the onerous task of critically evaluating many of the tests described. Finally, thanks are due to Dr B. Abernethy and Mr D. Spender, Basingstoke, England for help in preparing the text, and to Mr M. J. Lessiter, Birmingham, England for help with the illustrations of spot tests and thin-layer chromatography plates.

Introduction

After a brief introduction to the apparatus, reference compounds and reagents needed for an analytical toxicology laboratory (section 1), the manual covers a number of general topics, namely, clinical toxicology (section 2), clinical chemistry and haematology in relation to clinical toxicology (section 3), practical aspects of analytical toxicology (section 4), sample collection and storage, and qualitative poisons screening (section 5). Then, in a series of monographs (section 6), qualitative tests and some quantitative methods are described for 113 specific poisons or groups of poisons. Each monograph also includes some information on clinical interpretation.

The practical sections of the manual have been designed to be followed at the bench so that full experimental details of a test for a particular substance are often given, especially in the monographs (section 6), even though these same details may be repeated elsewhere in another context.

The tests described in sections 5 and 6 have been restricted to those that can be expected to produce reliable results within the limitations described, and that can be performed using relatively simple apparatus. Where appropriate, tests applicable to powders, tablets or other items found with or near the patient (scene residues) and to biological fluids are also included. Additional simple tests for specified pharmaceuticals are given in other World Health Organization publications.[a] However, these are designed to test the identity and in some cases stability of specific, relatively pure compounds and little consideration is given to, for example, purification procedures, sensitivity and sources of interference.

Primary references to particular methods have not been given, in order to simplify presentation and also because many tests have been modified over the years, so that reference back to the original paper could cause confusion. However, much of the information given in the manual can be found in the references listed in the Bibliography (p. 234). An attempt has been made to assess the sensitivity (detection limit) of all the qualitative tests given in the monographs (section 6). However, as

---

[a] *Basic tests for pharmaceutical substances.* Geneva, WHO, 1986; *Basic tests for pharmaceutical dosage forms.* Geneva, WHO, 1991.

with description of colour, such assessments are always to some extent subjective. In addition, the sensitivity of some tests, such as those involving solvent extraction, can usually be varied by taking more (or less) sample. These points emphasize the importance of analysing known negative (control) and positive (reference) samples alongside every specimen (see section 4.1.5).

Many of the terms used in this manual are defined in the Glossary (p. 237) and a list of reference compounds and reagents is provided (Annex 1).

Système internationale (International System; SI) mass units (mg/l, μg/l, etc.) have been used throughout to express concentrations of drugs and other poisons. There is a tendency to use SI molar units (mmol/l, μmol/l, etc.) for this purpose, but this can cause unnecessary confusion and has no clear advantage in analytical toxicology, provided that the exact chemical form of a substance is specified. SI mass/molar unit conversion factors for some common poisons are given in Annex 2. In some cases, SI mass units have also been used to express reagent concentrations, but it should be borne in mind that it is often sensible to prepare quantities of reagent smaller than one litre (100 ml, for example), especially for infrequently used tests.

For convenience, trivial or common chemical names have been used throughout the text; where necessary, IUPAC equivalents are given in the index. International nonproprietary names are used in the text for drugs; common synonyms are listed in the index.

1

Apparatus and reagents

1.1 Apparatus

Analytical toxicology services can be provided in clinical biochemistry laboratories that serve a local hospital or accident and emergency unit (of the type described in the WHO document *Laboratory services at the primary health care level*).[a] In addition to basic laboratory equipment, some specialized apparatus, such as that for thin-layer chromatography, ultraviolet and visible spectrophotometry and microdiffusion, is needed (Table 1). A continuous mains electricity supply is not essential.

No reference has been made to the use of more complex techniques, such as gas-liquid and high-performance liquid chromatography, atomic absorption spectrophotometry or immunoassays, even if simple methods are not available for particular compounds. Although such techniques are more selective and sensitive than many simple methods, there are a number of factors, in addition to operator expertise, that have to be considered before they can be used in individual laboratories. For example, the standards of quality (purity or cleanliness) of laboratory reagents and glassware and of consumable items such as solvents and gases needs to be considerably higher than for the tests described in this manual if reliable results are to be obtained.

Additional complications, which may not be apparent when instrument purchase is contemplated, include the need to ensure a regular supply of essential consumables (gas chromatographic septa, injection syringes, chromatography columns, solvent filters, chart or integrator paper, recorder ink or fibre-tip pens) and spare or additional parts (detector lamps, injection loops, column packing materials). The instruments must be properly maintained, which will usually require regular visits from the manufacturer's representative or agent. Indeed, such visits may need to be more frequent in developing countries, since the operating conditions (temperature, humidity, dust) can be more severe than those encountered elsewhere.

Some drug-testing facilities are now available in kit form. For example, there are standardized thin-layer chromatography (TLC) drug

---

[a] Unpublished document WHO/LAB/87.2. Available on request from Health Laboratory Technology and Blood Safety, World Health Organization, 1211 Geneva 27, Switzerland.

1

Table 1. Summary of basic equipment required for toxicological analyses

Reliable, regularly serviced and calibrated laboratory balances (top-pan and analytical) (section 4.1.3.)

Bench-top centrifuge (electrical or hand-driven) for separating blood samples and solvent extracts (section 4.3.2)

Vortex-mixer or other form of mechanical or hand-driven shaker such as a rotary mixer (section 4.3.2)

Water-bath and (electrical) heating block

Spirit lamp or butane gas burner

Refrigerator (electrical or evaporative) for storing standards/samples

pH meter

Range of automatic and semi-automatic pipettes (section 4.1.3)

Low-power, polarizing microscope

An adequate supply of laboratory glassware, including volumetric apparatus, and adequate cleaning facilities (section 4.1.5)

A supply of chemically pure water (section 4.1.4)

A supply of compressed air or nitrogen

A supply of thin-layer chromatography plates or facilities for preparing such plates (section 4.4.1)

Facilities for developing and visualizing thin-layer chromatograms, including an ultraviolet lamp (254 nm and 366 nm) and a fume cupboard or hood (section 4.4.4)

Single-beam or dual-beam ultraviolet/visible spectrophotometer and associated cells (section 4.5.2)

Conway microdiffusion apparatus (section 4.3.3)

Porcelain spotting tile (section 4.2)

Modified Gutzeit apparatus (section 6.6)

screening systems, which have the advantage that the plates are dipped or otherwise exposed to visualization reagents, and not sprayed, so that a fume cupboard or hood (see section 4.4.4) is not required. In addition, the interpretation of results is assisted by a compendium of annotated colour photographs. However, as with conventional TLC systems, interpretation can be difficult, especially if more than one compound is present. Further, the availability of the system and its associated consumables cannot be guaranteed.

Similarly, immunoassay kits are relatively simple to use, although problems can arise in practice, especially in the interpretation of results. Moreover, they are aimed primarily at the therapeutic drug monitoring and drug abuse testing markets and, as such, have limited direct application in clinical toxicology.

1.2 Reference compounds and reagents

A list of the reference compounds and reagents needed in a basic analytical toxicology laboratory is given in Annex 1. A supply of relatively pure compounds for use as reference standards is essential if reliable results are to be obtained. However, expensive reference compounds of a very high degree of purity, such as those marketed for use as pharmaceutical quality control standards, are not normally needed. Some drugs, such as barbital, caffeine and salicylic acid, and many inorganic and organic chemicals and solvents are available as laboratory reagents with an adequate degree of purity through normal laboratory chemical suppliers. Small quantities of a number of controlled drugs and some metabolites can be obtained from: Narcotics Laboratory Section, United Nations Vienna International Centre, P.O. Box 500, A-1400 Vienna, Austria.

It may be difficult to obtain small quantities (100 mg–1 g) of other drugs, pesticides, and their metabolites in pure form. Nevertheless, an attempt should be made to build up a reference collection or library (see Annex 1) without waiting for individual poisons to be found in patient samples. Such a reference collection is a valuable resource, and it should be stored under conditions that ensure safety, security and stability. If the pure compound cannot be obtained, then a pharmaceutical or other formulation is often the next best thing, and purification sufficient for at least a qualitative analysis can often be achieved by solvent extraction followed by recovery of the compound of interest (see section 4.1.2).

Although the apparatus required to perform the tests described in this manual is relatively simple, several unusual laboratory reagents are needed in order to be able to perform all of the tests described. Whenever possible, the shelf-life (stability) of individual compounds and reagents and any special precautions required in handling have been indicated in the text.

3

2

Clinical aspects of analytical toxicology

The trained analytical toxicologist can play a useful role in the management of patients poisoned with drugs or other chemicals. However, optimal analytical performance is only possible when the clinical aspects of the diagnosis and treatment of such patients are understood. The analyst must therefore have a basic knowledge of emergency medicine and intensive care, and must be able to communicate with clinicians. In addition, a good understanding of pharmacology and toxicology and some knowledge of active elimination procedures and the use of antidotes are desirable. This chapter aims to provide some of the basic information required.

2.1 Diagnosis of acute poisoning

2.1.1 Establishing a diagnosis

When acute poisoning is suspected, the clinician needs to ask a number of questions in order to establish a diagnosis. In the case of an unconscious (comatose) patient, the circumstances in which the patient was found and whether any tablet bottles or other containers (scene residues) were present can be important. If the patient is awake, he or she should be questioned about the presence of poisons in the home or workplace. The patient's past medical history (including drugs prescribed and any psychiatric illness), occupation and hobbies may also be relevant, since they may indicate possible access to specific poisons.

Physical examination of the patient may indicate the poison or class of poison involved. The clinical features associated with some common poisons are listed in Table 2. For example, the combination of pin-point pupils, hypersalivation, incontinence and respiratory depression suggests poisoning with a cholinesterase inhibitor such as an organophosphorus pesticide. However, the value of this approach is limited if a number of poisons with different actions have been absorbed. Moreover, many drugs have similar effects on the body, while some clinical features may be the result of secondary effects such as anoxia. Thus, if a patient is admitted with depressed respiration and pin-point pupils, this strongly suggests poisoning with an opioid such as dextropropoxyphene or morphine. However, if the pupils are dilated, then other hypnotic drugs

Table 2. Acute poisoning: clinical features associated with specific poisons

Clinical feature	Poison
Central nervous system	
Ataxia	Bromides, carbamazepine, ethanol, hypnotics/sedatives, phenytoin, thallium
Coma	Alcohols, hypnotics/sedatives, opioids, tranquillizers, many other compounds
Convulsions	Amitriptyline and other tricyclic antidepressants, orphenadrine, strychnine, theophylline
Respiratory tract	
Respiratory depression	Alcohols, hypnotics/sedatives, opioids, tranquillizers, many other compounds
Pulmonary oedema	Acetylsalicylic acid, chlorophenoxy herbicides, irritant (non-cardiogenic) gases, opioids, organic solvents, paraquat
Hyperpnoea	Acetysalicylic acid, ethylene glycol, hydroxybenzonitrile herbicides, isoniazid, methanol, pentachlorophenol
Heart and circulation	
Tachycardia	Anticholinergics, sympathomimetics
Bradycardia	Cholinergics, β-blockers, digoxin, opioids
Hypertension	Anticholinergics, sympathomimetics
Hypotension	Ethanol, hypnotics/sedatives, opioids, tranquillizers, many other compounds
Arrhythmias	β-Blockers, chloroquine, cyanide, digoxin, phenothiazines, quinidine, theophylline, tricyclic antidepressants
Eyes	
Miosis	Carbamate pesticides, opioids, organophosphorus pesticides, phencyclidine, phenothiazines
Mydriasis	Amfetamine, atropine, cocaine, tricyclic antidepressants
Nystagmus	Carbamazepine, ethanol, phenytoin
Body temperature	
Hyperthermia	Acetylsalicylic acid, dinitrophenol pesticides, hydroxybenzonitrile herbicides, pentachlorophenol, procainamide, quinidine
Hypothermia	Carbon monoxide, ethanol, hypnotics/sedatives, opioids, phenothiazines, tricyclic antidepressants
Skin, hair and nails	
Acne	Bromides, organochlorine pesticides
Hair loss	Thallium

5

Table 2 (contd.)

Clinical feature	Poison
Gastrointestinal tract	
Hypersalivation	Cholinesterase inhibitors, strychnine
Dry mouth	Atropine, opioids, phenothiazines, tricyclic anti-depressants
Constipation	Lead, opioids, thallium
Diarrhoea	Arsenic, cholinesterase inhibitors, laxatives
Gastrointestinal bleeding	Acetylsalicylic acid, caustic compounds (strong acids/bases), coumarin anticoagulants, indo-metacin
Liver damage	*Amanita* toxins, carbon tetrachloride, paraceta-mol, phosphorus (white)
Urogenital tract	
Urinary retention	Atropine, opioids, tricyclic antidepressants
Incontinence	Carbamate pesticides, organophosphorus pesti-cides
Kidney damage	*Amanita* toxins, cadmium, carbon tetrachloride, ethylene glycol, mercury, paracetamol

such as glutethimide may be present, or cerebral damage may have occurred as a result of hypoxia secondary to respiratory depression.

Diagnoses other than poisoning must also be considered. For example, coma can be caused by a cerebrovascular accident or uncontrolled diabetes as well as poisoning. The availability of the results of urgent biochemical and haematological tests is obviously important in these circumstances (see section 3). Finally, poisoning with certain compounds may be misdiagnosed, especially if the patient presents in the later stages of the episode. Examples include: cardiorespiratory arrest (cyanide), hepatitis (carbon tetrachloride, paracetamol), diabetes (hypoglycaemics, including ethanol in young children), paraesthesia (thallium), progressive pneumonitis (paraquat) and renal failure (ethylene glycol).

2.1.2 Classification of coma

Loss of consciousness (coma) is common in acute poisoning, especially if central nervous system (CNS) depressants are involved. A simple system, the Edinburgh scale (see Table 3), is often used to classify the depth or grade of coma of poisoned patients. This system has the advantage that the severity of an episode can be easily described in conversation with laboratory staff and with, for example, poisons information services that may be consulted for advice.

Table 3. Classification of depth of coma using the Edinburgh Scale

Grade of coma	Clinical features
1	Patient drowsy but responds to verbal commands
2	Patient unconscious but responds to minimal stimuli (for example, shaking, shouting)
3	Patient unconscious and responds only to painful stimuli (for example, rubbing the sternum)
4	Patient unconscious with no response to any stimuli

2.2 Treatment of acute poisoning

2.2.1 *General measures*

When acute poisoning is suspected, essential symptomatic and supportive measures are often taken before the diagnosis is confirmed. If the poison has been inhaled, the patient should first be removed from the contaminated environment. If skin contamination has occurred, contaminated clothing should be removed and the skin washed with an appropriate fluid, usually water. In adult patients, gastric aspiration and lavage (stomach washout) are often performed, if the poison has been ingested, to minimize the risk of continued absorption. Similarly, in children emesis can be induced by the oral administration of syrup of ipecacuanha (ipecac). The absorption of any residue remaining after gastric lavage can be minimized by leaving a high dose of activated charcoal in the stomach. The role of gavage and induced emesis in preventing absorption is currently being examined, as is the effectiveness of a single dose of activated charcoal. However, repeated oral administration of activated charcoal appears to be effective in enhancing elimination of certain poisons. Oral charcoal should **not** be given when oral administration of a protective agent, such as methionine following paracetamol overdosage, is contemplated.

Subsequently, most patients can be treated successfully using supportive care alone. In severely poisoned patients, this may include intravenous administration of anticonvulsants such as diazepam (see benzodiazepines) or clomethiazole, or of antiarrhythmics such as lidocaine, all of which may be detected if a toxicological analysis is performed later. Lidocaine is also used as a topical anaesthetic and is often found in urine as a result of incidental administration during urinary tract catheterization. Drugs or other compounds may also be given during investigative procedures such as lumbar puncture.

Specific therapeutic procedures, such as antidotal and active elimination therapy are sometimes indicated. The results of either a qualitative

7

or a quantitative toxicological analysis may be required before some treatments are commenced because they are not without risk to the patient. In general, specific therapy is only started when the nature and/or the amount of the poison(s) involved are known.

2.2.2 *Antidotes/protective agents*

Antidotes or protective agents are only available for a limited number of poisons (see Table 4). Controversy surrounds the use of some antidotes, such as those used to treat cyanide poisoning, while others are themselves potentially toxic and should be used with care. Lack of response

Table 4. Some antidotes and protective agents used to treat acute poisoning[a]

Antidote/agent	Indication
Acetylcysteine	Paracetamol
Atropine	Carbamate pesticides, organophosphorus pesticides
Deferoxamine	Aluminium, iron
DMSA[b]	Antimony, arsenic, bismuth, cadmium, lead, mercury
DMPS[c]	Copper, lead, mercury (elemental and inorganic)
Ethanol	Ethylene glycol, methanol
Antigen-binding (F_{ab}) antibody fragments	Digoxin
Flumazenil	Benzodiazepines
Methionine	Paracetamol
Methylene blue	Oxidizing agents (chlorates, nitrites, etc.)
Naloxone	Opioids (codeine, pethidine, morphine, etc.)
Obidoxime chloride (or pralidoxime iodide)	Organophosphorus pesticides (contraindicated with carbamate pesticides)
Oxygen	Carbon monoxide, cyanide
Physostigmine	Atropine
Phytomenadione (vitamin K_1)	Coumarin anticoagulants, indanedione anticoagulants
Potassium	Theophylline, barium
Protamine sulfate	Heparin
Prussian blue[d]	Thallium
Pyridoxine (vitamin B_6)	Isoniazid
Sodium calcium edetate	Lead, zinc

[a] Information on specific antidotes is given in the IPCS/CEC Evaluation of Antidotes Series; see Bibliography, p. 234.

[b] Dimercaptosuccinic acid

[c] Dimercaptopropanesulfonate

[d] Potassium ferrihexacyanoferrate

to a particular antidote does not necessarily indicate the absence of a particular type of poison. For example, the opioid antagonist naloxone will rapidly and completely reverse coma due to opioids such as morphine and codeine without risk to the patient, except that an acute withdrawal response may be precipitated in dependent subjects. However, a lack of response does not always mean that opioids are not present, since another, non-opioid, drug may be the cause of coma, too little naloxone may have been given, or hypoxic brain damage may have followed a cardiorespiratory or respiratory arrest.

2.2.3 *Active elimination therapy*

There are four main methods of enhancing elimination of the poison from the systemic circulation: repeated oral activated charcoal; forced diuresis with alteration of urine pH; peritoneal dialysis and haemodialysis; and haemoperfusion.

The systemic clearance of compounds such as barbiturates, carbamazepine, quinine and theophylline (and possibly also salicylic acid and its derivatives) can be enhanced by giving oral activated charcoal at intervals of 4–6 hours until clinical recovery is apparent. To reduce transit time and thus reabsorption of the poison, the charcoal is often given together with a laxative. This procedure has the advantage of being totally noninvasive but is less effective if the patient has a paralytic ileus resulting from the ingestion of, for example, phenobarbital. Care must also be taken to avoid pulmonary aspiration in patients without a gag reflex or in those with a depressed level of consciousness.

The aim of forced diuresis is to enhance urinary excretion of the poison by increasing urine volume per unit of time. It is achieved by means of intravenous administration of a compatible fluid. Nowadays, forced diuresis is almost always combined with manipulation of urine pH. Renal elimination of weak acids such as chlorophenoxy herbicides and salicylates can be increased by the intravenous administration of sodium bicarbonate. This can also protect against systemic toxicity by favouring partition into aqueous compartments such as blood. Indeed, alkalinization alone can be as effective as traditional forced alkaline diuresis, and has the advantage that the risk of complications resulting from fluid overload, such as cerebral or pulmonary oedema and electrolyte disturbance, is minimized. However, the pK of the poison must be such that renal elimination can be enhanced by alterations in urinary pH within the physiological range. It is also important to monitor urine pH carefully to ensure that the desired change has been achieved. Acidification of urine was thought to enhance the clearance of weak bases such as amfetamine, procyclidine and quinine, but this is no longer generally accepted.

Dialysis and haemoperfusion remove the poison directly from the circulation. In haemodialysis, blood is passed over a membrane which is in contact with the aqueous compartment in an artificial kidney, while in peritoneal dialysis an appropriate fluid is infused into the peritoneal cavity and then drained some 2–4 hours later. In haemoperfusion, blood is pumped through a cartridge of adsorbent material (coated activated charcoal or Amberlite XAD-4 resin). Haemodialysis is preferred for water-soluble substances such as ethanol, and haemoperfusion for lipophilic poisons such as short-acting barbiturates, which have a high affinity for coated charcoal or Amberlite XAD-4 resin. The decision to use dialysis or haemoperfusion should be based on the clinical condition of the patient, the properties of the poison ingested and its concentration in plasma. Haemodialysis and haemoperfusion are only effective when the volume of distribution of the poison is small, i.e., relative volume of distribution less than 5 l/kg.

2.3 The role of the clinical toxicology laboratory

Most poisoned patients can be treated successfully without any contribution from the laboratory other than routine clinical biochemistry and haematology. This is particularly true for those cases where there is no

Table 5. Steps in undertaking an analytical toxicological investigation

Step	Action
Pre-analytical phase	
1.	Obtain details of current admission, including any circumstantial evidence of poisoning and results of biochemical and haematological investigations (see section 3).
2.	Obtain patient's medical history, if available, ensure access to the appropriate sample(s), and decide the priorities for the analysis.
Analytical phase	
3.	Perform the agreed analyses.
Post-analytical phase	
4.	Interpret the results and discuss them with the clinician looking after the patient.
5.	Perform additional analyses, if indicated, on the original samples or on further samples from the patient.

Table 6. Interpretation of emergency toxicological analyses

Poison	Concentration[a] associated with serious toxicity	Treatment
1. *Protective therapy*		
Paracetamol	200 mg/l at 4 h after ingestion 30 mg/l at 15 h after ingestion	Acetylcysteine or methionine
Methanol	0.5 g/l	Ethanol
Ethylene glycol	0.5 g/l	
Thallium	0.2 mg/l (urine)	Prussian blue[b]
2. *Chelation therapy*		
Iron	5 mg/l (serum)	Deferoxamine
Aluminium	50–250 µg/l (serum)	
Lead	1 mg/l (whole blood, adults)	DMSA[c]/DMPS[d]/ Sodium calcium edetate
Cadmium	20 µg/l (whole blood)	DMSA
Mercury	100 µg/l (whole blood)	DMSA/DMPS
Arsenic	200 µg/l (whole blood)	DMSA
3. *Active elimination therapy*		
Acetylsalicylic acid (as salicylate)	900 mg/l at 6 hours after ingestion 450 mg/l at 24 hours after ingestion	Alkaline diuresis
Phenobarbital	200 mg/l	
Barbital	300 mg/l	
Chlorophenoxy herbicides	500 mg/l	
Ethanol	5 g/l	Peritoneal dialysis or haemodialysis
Methanol	0.5 g/l	
Ethylene glycol	0.5 g/l	
Phenobarbital	200 mg/l	
Barbital	300 mg/l	
Acetylsalicylic acid (as salicylate)	900 mg/l at 6 h, 450 mg/l at 24 h	
Lithium	14 mg/l	
Phenobarbital	100 mg/l	Charcoal haemoperfusion
Barbital	200 mg/l	
Other barbiturates	50 mg/l	
Theophylline	100 mg/l	

[a] In plasma, unless otherwise specified.

[b] Potassium ferrihexacyanoferrate

[c] Dimercaptosuccinic acid

[d] Dimercaptopropanesulfonate

doubt about the poison involved and when the results of a quantitative analysis would not affect therapy. However, toxicological analyses can play a useful role if the diagnosis is in doubt, the administration of antidotes or protective agents is contemplated, or the use of active elimination therapy is being considered. The analyst's dealings with a case of poisoning are usually divided into pre-analytical, analytical and post-analytical phases (see Table 5).

Practical aspects of the collection, transport, and storage of the samples appropriate to a particular analysis are given in section 5 and in the monographs (section 6). Tests for any poisons that the patient is thought to have taken and for which specific therapy is available will normally be given priority over coma screening. This topic is discussed fully in section 5 where a poisons screen is also outlined. Tests for individual poisons or groups of poisons are given in section 6.

Finally, an attempt must always be made to correlate the laboratory findings with clinical observations. In order to do so, some knowledge of the toxicological effects of the substances in question is required (see Table 2). Additional information on individual poisons is given in the monographs (section 6) and in the clinical toxicology textbooks listed in the Bibliography. Some instances where treatment might be influenced by the results of toxicological analyses are listed in Table 6.

3
General laboratory findings in clinical toxicology

Many clinical laboratory tests can be helpful in the diagnosis of acute poisoning and in assessing prognosis. Those discussed here (which are listed in Table 7) are likely to be the most useful, although only the largest laboratories may be able to offer all of them on an emergency basis. More specialized tests may be appropriate depending on the clinical condition of the patient, the circumstantial evidence of poisoning and the past medical history. Tests used in monitoring supportive treatment are not considered here; details of such tests can be found in standard clinical chemistry textbooks (see Bibliography, p. 234).

3.1 Biochemical tests

3.1.1 Blood glucose

Marked hypoglycaemia often results from overdosage with insulin, sulfonylureas, such as tolbutamide, or other antidiabetic drugs. Hypoglycaemia may also complicate severe poisoning with a number of agents including iron salts and certain fungi, and may follow ingestion of acetylsalicylic acid, ethanol (especially in children or fasting adults) and paracetamol if liver failure ensues. Hypoglycin is a potent hypoglycaemic agent found in unripe ackee fruit (*Blighia sapida*) and is responsible for Jamaican vomiting sickness. Hyperglycaemia is a less common complication of poisoning than hypoglycaemia, but has been reported after overdosage with acetylsalicylic acid, salbutamol and theophylline.

3.1.2 Electrolytes, blood gases and pH

Coma resulting from overdosage with hypnotic, sedative, neuroleptic or opioid drugs is often characterized by hypoxia and respiratory acidosis. Unless appropriate treatment is instituted, however, a mixed acid–base disturbance with metabolic acidosis will supervene. In contrast, overdosage with salicylates such as acetylsalicylic acid initially causes hyperventilation and respiratory alkalosis, which may progress to the mixed metabolic acidosis and hypokalaemia characteristic of severe poisoning. Hypokalaemia and metabolic acidosis are also features of theophylline and salbutamol overdosage. Hypokalaemia occurs in acute

Table 7. Some laboratory tests likely to be useful in clinical toxicology

Fluid	Qualitative test	Quantitative test
Urine	Colour (haematuria, myoglobinuria)	Relative density
		pH
	Smell	
	Turbidity	
	Crystalluria	
Blood	Colour (oxygenation)	pCO_2, pO_2, pH
		Glucose
		Prothrombin time
		Carboxyhaemoglobin
		Methaemoglobin
		Erythrocyte volume fraction (haematocrit)
		Leukocyte count
		Platelet count
Plasma	Lipaemia	Bilirubin
		Electrolytes (Na^+, K^+, Ca^{2+}, Cl^-, HCO_3^-)
		Lactate
		Osmolality
		Plasma enzymes[a]
		Cholinesterase

[a] Lactate dehydrogenase, aspartate aminotransferase, alanine aminotransferase, creatine kinase

barium poisoning, but severe acute overdosage with digoxin gives rise to hyperkalaemia.

Toxic substances or their metabolites, which inhibit key steps in intermediary metabolism, are likely to cause metabolic acidosis owing to the accumulation of organic acids, notably lactate. In severe poisoning of this nature, the onset of metabolic acidosis can be rapid and prompt corrective treatment is vital. Measurement of the serum or plasma anion gap can be helpful in distinguishing toxic metabolic acidosis from that associated with nontoxic faecal or renal loss of bicarbonate. The anion gap is usually calculated as the difference between the sodium concentration and the sum of the chloride and bicarbonate concentrations. It is normally about 10 mmol/l and also corresponds to the sum of plasma potassium, calcium and magnesium concentrations. This value is little changed in nontoxic metabolic acidosis. However, in metabolic acidosis resulting from severe poisoning with carbon monoxide, cyanide, ethylene glycol, methanol, fluoroacetates, paraldehyde or acetylsalicylic acid, the anion gap may exceed 15 mmol/l. Toxic metabolic acidosis may also occur in severe poisoning with iron, ethanol, paracetamol, isoniazid, phenformin and theophylline.

Other acid–base or electrolyte disturbances occur in many types of poisoning for a variety of reasons. Such disturbances are sometimes simple to monitor and to interpret, but are more often complex. The correct interpretation of serial measurements requires a detailed knowledge of the therapy administered. Hyperkalaemia or hypernatraemia occurs in iatrogenic, accidental or deliberate overdosage with potassium or sodium salts. The consequences of electrolyte imbalances depend on many factors, including the state of hydration, the integrity of renal function, and concomitant changes in sodium, calcium, magnesium, chloride and phosphate metabolism. Hyponatraemia can result from many causes, including water intoxication, inappropriate loss of sodium, or impaired excretion of water by the kidney. Hypocalcaemia can occur in ethylene glycol poisoning owing to sequestration of calcium by oxalic acid.

3.1.3 Plasma osmolality

The normal osmolality of plasma (280–295 mOsm/kg) is largely accounted for by sodium, urea and glucose. Unusually high values (> 310 mOsm/kg) can occur in pathological conditions such as gross proteinaemia or severe dehydration where the effective proportion of water in plasma is reduced. However, large increases in plasma osmolality may follow the absorption of osmotically active poisons (especially methanol, ethanol or propan-2-ol) in relatively large amounts. Ethylene glycol, acetone and some other organic substances with a low relative molecular mass are also osmotically active in proportion to their molar concentration (see Table 8).

Although the measurement of plasma osmolality can give useful information, interpretation can be difficult. For example, there may be

Table 8. Effect of some common poisons on plasma osmolality

Compound	Plasma osmolality increase (mOsm/kg) for 0.01 g/l	Analyte concentration (g/l) corresponding to 1 mOsm/kg increase in plasma osmolality
Acetone	0.18	0.055
Ethanol	0.22	0.046
Ethylene glycol	0.20	0.050
Methanol	0.34	0.029
Propan-2-ol	0.17	0.059

secondary dehydration, as in overdosage with salicylates, ethanol may have been taken together with a more toxic, osmotically active substance, or enteral or parenteral therapy may have involved the administration of large amounts of sugar alcohols (mannitol, sorbitol) or formulations containing glycerol or propylene glycol.

3.1.4 Plasma enzymes

Shock, coma, and convulsions are often associated with nonspecific increases in the plasma or serum activities of enzymes (lactate dehydrogenase, aspartate aminotransferase, alanine aminotransferase) commonly measured to detect damage to the major organs. Usually the activities increase over a period of a few days and slowly return to normal values. Such changes are of little diagnostic or prognostic value.

The plasma activities of liver enzymes may increase rapidly after absorption of toxic doses of substances that can cause liver necrosis, notably paracetamol, carbon tetrachloride, and copper salts. It may take several weeks for values to return to normal. The plasma activities of the aminotransferases may be higher than normal in patients on chronic therapy with drugs such as valproic acid, and serious hepatotoxicity may develop in a small proportion of patients. Chronic ethanol abuse is usually associated with increased plasma γ-glutamyltransferase activity.

In very severe poisoning, especially if a prolonged period of coma, convulsions or shock has occurred, there is likely to be clinical or subclinical muscle injury associated with rhabdomyolysis and disseminated intravascular coagulation. Such damage can also occur as a result of chronic parenteral abuse of psychotropic drugs. Frank rhabdomyolysis is characterized by high serum aldolase or creatine kinase activities together with myoglobinuria. This can be detected by *o*-toluidine-based reagents or test strips, provided there is no haematuria. In serious cases of poisoning, for example with strychnine, myoglobinuria together with high serum or plasma potassium, uric acid and phosphate concentrations may indicate the onset of acute kidney failure.

3.1.5 Cholinesterase activity

Systemic toxicity from carbamate and organophosphorus pesticides is due largely to the inhibition of acetylcholinesterase at nerve synapses. Cholinesterase, derived initially from the liver, is also present in plasma, but inhibition of plasma cholinesterase is not thought to be physiologically important. It should be emphasized that cholinesterase and acetylcholinesterase are different enzymes: plasma cholinesterase can be almost completely inhibited while erythrocyte acetylcholinesterase still possesses 50% activity. This relative inhibition varies between compounds and with the route of absorption and depending on whether exposure has been acute, chronic or acute-on-chronic. In addition, the rate at which cholinesterase inhibition is reversed depends on whether the inhibition was caused by carbamate or organophosphorus pesticides.

In practice, plasma cholinesterase is a useful indicator of exposure to organophosphorus compounds or carbamates, and a normal plasma cholinesterase activity effectively excludes acute poisoning by these compounds. The difficulty lies in deciding whether a low activity is indeed due to poisoning or to some other physiological, pharmacological or genetic cause. The diagnosis can sometimes be assisted by detection of a poison or metabolite in a body fluid, but the simple methods available are relatively insensitive (see sections 6.19 and 6.80). Alternatively pralidoxime, used as an antidote in poisoning with organophosphorus pesticides (see Table 4), can be added to a portion of the test plasma or serum *in vitro* (section 6.30). Pralidoxime antagonises the effect of organophosphorus compounds on cholinesterase. Therefore if cholinesterase activity is maintained in the pralidoxime-treated portion of the sample but inhibited in the portion not treated with pralidoxime, this provides strong evidence that an organophosphorus compound is present.

Erythrocyte (red cell) acetylcholinesterase activity can be measured, but this enzyme is membrane-bound and the apparent activity depends on the methods used in solubilization and separation from residual plasma cholinesterase. At present there is no standard procedure. Erythrocyte acetylcholinesterase activity also depends on the rate of erythropoiesis. Newly formed erythrocytes have a high activity which diminishes with time. Hence erythrocyte acetylcholinesterase activity is a function of the number and age of the cell population. However, low activities of both plasma cholinesterase and erythrocyte acetylcholinesterase is strongly suggestive of poisoning with either organophosphorus or carbamate pesticides.

3.2 Haematological tests

3.2.1 Blood clotting

Prolonged prothrombin time is a valuable early indicator of liver damage in poisoning with metabolic toxins such as paracetamol. The prothrombin time and other measures of blood clotting are likely to be abnormal in acute poisoning with rodenticides such as coumarin anticoagulants, and after overdosage with heparin or other anticoagulants. Coagulopathies may also occur as a side-effect of antibiotic therapy. The occurrence of disseminated intravascular coagulation together with rhabdomyolysis in severe poisoning cases (prolonged coma, convulsions, shock) has already been discussed (section 3.1.4).

3.2.2 *Carboxyhaemoglobin and methaemoglobin*

Measurement of blood carboxyhaemoglobin can be used to assess the severity of acute carbon monoxide poisoning and chronic dichloromethane poisoning. However, carboxyhaemoglobin is dissociated rapidly once the patient is removed from the contaminated atmosphere, especially if oxygen is administered, and the sample should therefore be obtained as soon as possible after admission. Even then, blood carboxyhaemoglobin concentrations tend to correlate poorly with clinical features of toxicity.

Methaemoglobin (oxidized haemoglobin) may be formed after overdosage with dapsone and oxidizing agents such as chlorates or nitrites, and can be induced by exposure to aromatic nitro compounds (such as nitrobenzene and aniline and some of its derivatives). The production of methaemoglobinaemia with intravenous sodium nitrite is a classical method of treating acute cyanide poisoning. Methaemoglobinaemia may be indicated by the presence of dark chocolate-coloured blood. Blood methaemoglobin can be measured but is unstable and results from stored samples are unreliable.

3.2.3 *Erythrocyte volume fraction (haematocrit)*

Acute or acute-on-chronic overdosage with iron salts, acetylsalicylic acid, indometacin, and other nonsteroidal anti-inflammatory drugs may cause gastrointestinal bleeding leading to anaemia. Anaemia may also result from chronic exposure to toxins that interfere with haem synthesis, such as lead, or induce haemolysis either directly (arsine, see arsenic) or indirectly because of glucose-6-phosphate dehydrogenase deficiency (chloroquine, primaquine, chloramphenicol, nitridazole, nitrofurantoin).

3.2.4 *Leukocyte count*

Increases in the leukocyte (white blood cell) count often occur in acute poisoning, for example, in response to an acute metabolic acidosis, resulting from ingestion of ethylene glycol or methanol, or secondary to hypostatic pneumonia following prolonged coma.

4

Practical aspects of analytical toxicology

It has been assumed that users of this manual will have some practical knowledge of clinical chemistry and be familiar with basic laboratory operations, including aspects of laboratory health and safety. However, some aspects of laboratory practice are particularly important if results are to be reliable and these are discussed in this section.

Many of the topics discussed here and in sections 5 and 6 (use of clinical specimens, samples and standards, pretreatment of samples, thin-layer chromatography, ultraviolet/visible spectrophotometry) are the subject of monographs in the Analytical Chemistry by Open Learning (ACOL) series. The material contained in those monographs is complementary to that given here, and the volumes will be useful to those without a background in analytical chemistry. Details of ACOL texts are given in the Bibliography (p. 234).

4.1 Laboratory management and practice

4.1.1 Health and safety in the laboratory

Many of the tests described in this manual entail the use of extremely toxic chemicals. The toxicity of some of them is not widely recognized (the ingestion of as little as 20–30 ml of the commonly used solvent methanol, for example, can cause serious toxicity in an adult). Some specific hazards have been highlighted, but many have been assumed to be self-evident — for example, strong acids and alkalis should **never** be stored together, strong acids or alkalis should always be added to water and **not** vice versa, organic solvents should **not** be heated over a naked flame but in a water-bath, and a fume cupboard or hood should **always** be used when organic solvents are evaporated or thin-layer chromatography plates are sprayed with visualization reagents.

Laboratory staff should be aware of local policies regarding health and safety and especially of regulations regarding the processing of potentially infective biological specimens. There should also be a written health and safety policy that is available to, and understood by, all staff, and there should be practical, written instructions on how to handle and dispose of biological samples, organic solvents and other hazardous or potentially hazardous substances. A health and safety officer should be appointed from among the senior laboratory staff with responsibility for the enforcement of this policy. Ideally, disposable plastic gloves and safety spectacles should be worn at all times in the laboratory. Details of the hazards associated with the use of particular chemicals and reagents can often be obtained from the supplier.

4.1.2 *Reagents and drug standards*

Chemicals obtained from a reputable supplier are normally graded as to purity (analytical reagent grade, general purpose reagent, laboratory reagent grade, etc.). The maximum limits of common or important impurities are often stated on the label, together with recommended storage conditions. Some chemicals readily absorb atmospheric water vapour and either remain solid (hygroscopic, for example the sodium salt of phenytoin) or enter solution (deliquescent, for example trichloroacetic acid — see section 6.24), and thus should be stored in a desiccator. Others (for example, sodium hydroxide) readily absorb atmospheric carbon dioxide either when solid or in solution, while phosphate buffer solutions are notorious for permitting the growth of bacteria (often visible as a cloudy precipitate).

Where chemicals or primary standards, such as drugs, are obtained from secondary sources, it is important to have some idea of the purity of the sample. Useful information can often be obtained by carrying out a simple thin-layer chromatographic analysis, and the ultraviolet spectrum can also be valuable. It is also possible to measure the absorbance of a solution of the drug and compare the result with tabulated specific absorbance values (the absorbance of a 1% (w/v) solution in a cell of 1-cm path length, see section 4.5.1). For example, the specific absorbances for the drug colchicine in ethanol are 730 and 350 at 243 nm and 425 nm, respectively. Thus, a 10 mg/l solution in ethanol should give absorbance readings of 0.73 and 0.35 at 243 nm and 425 nm, respectively, in a cell of 1-cm path length. However, this procedure does not rule out the presence of impurities with similar relative molecular masses and specific absorbance values.

4.1.3 *Balances and pipettes*

Balances for weighing reagents or standards and automatic and semi-automatic pipettes must be kept clean and checked for accuracy regularly. Semi-automatic pipettes are normally calibrated to measure aqueous fluids (relative density about 1), and should not be used for organic solvents or other solutions with relative densities or viscosities greatly different from those of water. Positive displacement pipettes should be used for very viscous fluids, such as whole blood. Accuracy can easily be tested by weighing or dispensing purified (distilled or deionized) water; the volumes of 1.0000 g of distilled water at different temperatures are given in Table 9. Low relative humidities may give rise to static electrical effects, particularly with plastic weighing boats, which can influence the weight recorded.

When preparing important reagents or primary standards, particular attention should be paid to the relative molecular masses (molecular weights) of salts and their degree of hydration (water of crystallization). A simple example is the preparation of a cyanide solution with a cyanide ion concentration of 50 mg/l. Potassium cyanide has a relative molecular mass of 65.1 while that of the cyanide ion is 26.0. A solution with a cyanide ion concentration of 50 mg/l is therefore equivalent to a potassium cyanide concentration of $50 \times 65.1/26.0$ mg/l, i.e., 125.2 mg/l. Particular care should be taken when weighing out primary calibration standards, and the final weight plus tare (weighing boat) weight should be recorded.

4.1.4 Chemically pure water

Tapwater or well water is likely to contain dissolved material which renders it unsuitable for laboratory use, so it is essential that any water used for the preparation of reagents or standard solutions is purified by distillation or deionization using a commercial ion-exchange process. The simplest procedure is distillation using an all-glass apparatus (glass distilled). The distillation should not be allowed to proceed too vigorously otherwise impurities may simply boil over into the distillate.

Table 9. Volume of 1.0000 g of distilled water at different temperatures

Temperature (°C)	Volume (ml)	Temperature (°C)	Volume (ml)
15	1.0020	24	1.0037
16	1.0021	25	1.0039
17	1.0023	26	1.0042
18	1.0025	27	1.0045
19	1.0026	28	1.0047
20	1.0028	29	1.0050
21	1.0030	30	1.0053
22	1.0032	31	1.0056
23	1.0034	32	1.0059

Potassium permanganate and sodium hydroxide (each at about 100 mg/l) added to the water to be distilled will oxidize or ionize volatile organic compounds or nitrogenous bases, and thus minimize contamination of the purified water. If highly purified water is required then water already distilled can be redistilled (double distilled). The pH of distilled water is usually about 4 because of the presence of dissolved carbon dioxide.

4.1.5 Quality assurance

Known positive and negative specimens should normally be analysed at the same time as the test sample. A negative control (blank) helps to ensure that false positives (owing to, for example, contaminated reagents or glassware) are not obtained. Equally, inclusion of a true positive serves to check that the reagents have been prepared properly and have maintained their stability. Suspected false positive tests should be repeated using glassware freshly cleaned with an organic solvent such as methanol and/or purified water. In general, all glassware, particularly test-tubes, should be rinsed in tapwater immediately after use. This should be followed by rigorous cleaning in warm laboratory detergent solution, then rinsing in tapwater and in purified water before air-drying. Badly contaminated glassware can be soaked initially in concentrated sulfuric acid (relative density 1.83) containing 100 g/litre potassium dichromate (acid/dichromate, chromic acid). However, this mixture is extremely dangerous, and treatment with a modern laboratory detergent is usually all that is needed.

Quantitative tests require even more vigilance to ensure accuracy and precision (reproducibility). When a new batch of a standard solution is prepared it is prudent to compare the results obtained in analysing a material of known concentration with those given by an earlier batch or an external source to ensure that errors have not been made in preparation. As in other areas of clinical laboratory practice, it is important to organize an internal quality control scheme for all quantitative procedures, and to participate in external quality assurance schemes whenever possible.

4.1.6 Recording and reporting results

All results should be recorded on laboratory worksheets together with the date, the name of the analyst, the name of the patient, and other relevant information, including the number and nature of the specimens received for analysis, and the tests performed. (An example of a laboratory worksheet is given in Fig. 3, page 39). It is advisable to allocate to each specimen a unique identifying number as it is received in the laboratory, and to use this number when referring to the tests performed using this specimen. Ultraviolet spectra, calibration graphs and other documents generated during an analysis should always be kept for a period of time after the results have been reported. The recording of results of colour tests and thin-layer chromatographic analyses is more difficult, and is discussed in subsequent sections. Doubtful or unusual results should always be discussed with senior staff. When reporting the results of tests in which no compounds were detected in plasma/serum or in urine, the limit of sensitivity of the test (detection limit) should always be known, at least to the laboratory, and the scope of generic tests (for example, for benzodiazepines or opioids) should be defined.

In analytical toxicology, SI mass units should be used to report the results of quantitative analyses. The femtogram (fg) $= 10^{-15}$ g, picogram (pg) $= 10^{-12}$ g, nanogram (ng) $= 10^{-9}$ g, microgram (μg) $= 10^{-6}$ g, milligram (mg) $= 10^{-3}$ g, gram (g) and kilogram (kg) $= 10^{3}$ g are the preferred units of mass, and the litre (l) is the preferred unit of volume. Other units of concentration, mg %, mg/dl, μg/ml and ppm (parts per million), are often encountered in the literature. It is useful to remember that: 1 mg/l $= 1$ ppm $= 1$ μg/ml $= 0.1$ mg % $= 0.1$ mg/dl.

Some clinical chemistry departments report analytical toxicology results in SI molar units (μmol/l, mmol/l, etc.). A list of conversion factors is given in Annex 2. This is an area with great potential for confusion, and care must be taken to ensure that the clinician is fully aware of the units in which quantitative results are reported.

4.2 Colour tests

Many drugs and other poisons, if present in sufficient concentration and in the absence of interfering compounds, give characteristic colours with appropriate reagents. Some of these tests are, for practical purposes, specific, but compounds containing similar functional groups will also react, and thus interference from other poisons, metabolites or contaminants is to be expected. Further complications are that colour description is very subjective, even in people with normal colour vision, while the colours produced usually vary in intensity or hue with concentration, and may also be unstable.

Many of these tests can be performed satisfactorily in clear glass test-tubes. However, use of a spotting tile (a white glazed porcelain tile with a number of shallow depressions or wells in its surface) gives a uniform background against which to assess any colours produced, and also minimizes the volumes of reagents and sample that need to be used. Colour tests feature prominently in the monographs (section 6), where common problems and sources of interference in particular tests are emphasized. When performing colour tests it is always important to analyse concurrently with the test sample:

(a) a reagent blank, i.e., an appropriate sample known **not** to contain the compound(s) of interest; if the test is to be performed on urine, then blank (analyte-free) urine should be used, otherwise water is adequate;

(b) a known positive sample at an appropriate concentration. If the test is to be performed on urine, then ideally urine from a patient or volunteer known to have taken the compound in question should be used. However, this is not always practicable and then spiked urine (blank urine to which a known amount of the compound under analysis has been added) should be used.

4.3 Pretreatment of samples

4.3.1 Introduction

Although many of the tests described in this manual can be performed directly on biological fluids or other aqueous solution, some form of sample pretreatment is often required. With plasma and serum, a simple form of pretreatment is protein precipitation by vortex-mixing with, for example, an aqueous solution of trichloroacetic acid, followed by centrifugation to produce a clear supernatant for analysis. Hydrolysis of some compounds, including possibly conjugated metabolites in urine (sulfates and glucuronides), either by heating with acid or by treatment with an enzyme preparation, is also employed. This either gives a reactive compound for the test (as with benzodiazepines and paracetamol) or enhances sensitivity (as with laxatives and morphine).

4.3.2 Solvent extraction

Liquid–liquid extraction of drugs and other lipophilic poisons from the specimen into an appropriate, water-immiscible, organic solvent, usually at a controlled pH, is widely used in analytical toxicology. Solvent extraction removes water and dissolved interfering compounds, and reduction in volume (by evaporation) of the extract before analysis provides a simple means of concentrating the compounds of interest and thus enhancing sensitivity.

Some form of mechanical mixing of the aqueous and organic phases is normally necessary. Of the methods available, vortex-mixing is the quickest and the most efficient for relatively small volumes. Rotary mixers capable of accepting tubes of up to 30 ml in volume are valuable for performing relatively large volume extracts of plasma/serum, urine, or stomach contents, and serve to minimize the risk of emulsion formation. Centrifugation in a bench-top centrifuge, again capable of accepting test-tubes of up to 30 ml in volume and attaining speeds of 2000–3000 rev/min, is normally effective in separating the phases so that the organic extract can be removed. Ideally, the centrifuge should have a sealed motor unit (which is flashproof) and tubes should be sealed to minimize both the risk of explosion from ignition of solvent vapour and the risks associated with centrifugation of infective specimens. Finally, filtration of the organic extract through silicone-treated phase-separating paper prevents contamination of the extract with small amounts of aqueous phase.

Commercial prebuffered extraction tubes (so-called solid-phase extraction) are now widely used for liquid–liquid extraction, especially in preparing urine extracts for drug screening (see section 5.2.3). Such tubes have the advantage that a wide range of basic compounds, including morphine, and weak acids, such as barbiturates, can be extracted in a single step. However, they are relatively expensive and cannot be re-used.

4.3.3 *Microdiffusion*

Microdiffusion is also a form of sample purification and relies on the liberation of a volatile compound (hydrogen cyanide in the case of cyanide salts) from the test solution held in one compartment of an enclosed system such as the specially constructed Conway apparatus (Fig. 1). The volatile compound is subsequently trapped using an appropriate reagent (sodium hydroxide solution in the case of hydrogen cyanide) held in a separate compartment.

The cells are normally allowed to stand for 2–5 hours at room temperature for the diffusion process to be completed. The analyte concentration is subsequently measured in a portion of the trapping solution either by spectrophotometry or by visual comparison with standards analysed concurrently in separate cells. The Conway apparatus is normally made from glass, but polycarbonate must be used with fluorides since hydrogen fluoride etches glass. The cover is often smeared with petroleum jelly or silicone grease to ensure an airtight seal. In order to carry out a quantitative assay at least eight cells are needed: one blank, three calibration samples, two test samples and two positive

Fig. 1. Conway microdiffusion apparatus

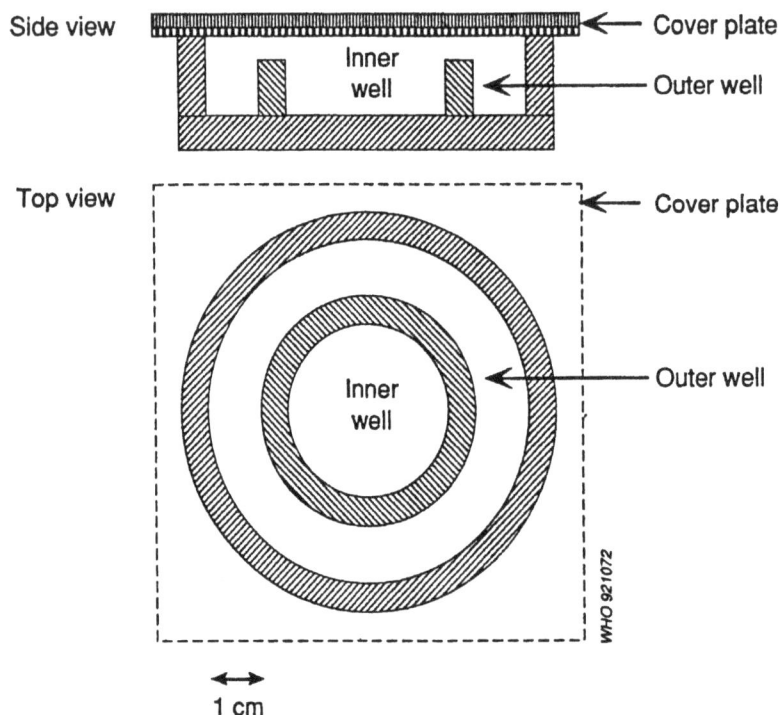

controls. It is important to clean the diffusion apparatus carefully after use, possibly using an acid/dichromate mixture (see section 4.1.5), rinsing it in distilled water before drying.

4.4 Thin-layer chromatography

Thin-layer chromatography (TLC) involves the movement by capillary action of a liquid phase (usually an organic solvent) through a thin, uniform layer of stationary phase (usually silica gel, SiO_2) held on a rigid or semi-rigid support, normally a glass, aluminium or plastic sheet or plate. Compounds are separated by partition between the mobile and stationary phases. TLC is relatively inexpensive and simple to perform, and can be a powerful qualitative technique when used together with some form of sample pretreatment, such as solvent extraction. However, some separations can be difficult to reproduce. The interpretation of results can also be very difficult, especially if a number of drugs or metabolites are present.

TLC of solvent extracts of urine, stomach contents or scene residues forms the basis of the drug screening procedure outlined in section 5.2.3, and is also recommended for the detection and identification of a number of compounds described in the monographs (section 6). TLC can also be used as a semiquantitative technique, as described in the monograph on coumarin anticoagulants (section 6.35).

The aim of this section is to provide practical information on the use of TLC in analytical toxicology. More general information on the theory and practice of TLC can be found in the references listed in the Bibliography (p. 234).

4.4.1 *Preparation of TLC plates*

The stationary phase is normally a uniform film (0.25 mm in thickness) of silica gel (average particle size 20 μm). Plates usually measure 20 × 20 cm, although smaller sizes can also be used. Some commercially available plates incorporate a fluorescent indicator, and this may be useful in locating spots prior to spraying with visualization reagents. Prior soaking of the plate in methanolic potassium hydroxide and drying may improve the chromatography of some basic compounds using certain solvent systems but, generally, addition of concentrated ammonium hydroxide (relative density 0.88) to the mobile phase has the same effect (section 5.2.3). High-performance TLC (HPTLC) plates have a smaller average particle size (5–10 μm) and greater efficiency than conventional plates. Reversed-phase plates, which have a hydrophobic moiety (usually C_2, C_8 or C_{18}) bonded to the silica matrix, are also available. However, HPTLC and reversed-phase plates are more expensive and have a lower sample capacity than conventional plates, and are not recommended for the procedures outlined in this manual.

TLC plates can be prepared in the laboratory from silica gel containing an appropriate binding agent and glass plates measuring 20 × 20 × 0.5 cm. It is important to ensure that the plates are clean and free from grease. The silica gel is first mixed with twice its own weight of water to form a slurry. The slurry is then quickly applied to the glass plate using a commercial spreader to form a film 0.25 mm in thickness. Small amounts of additives such as fluorescent markers can be included if required. The plates are dried in air and should be kept free of moisture prior to use. The quality of such home-made TLC plates should be carefully monitored; activation (i.e., heating at 100 °C for 30 minutes prior to use) may be helpful in maintaining performance. Dipping techniques, whereby glass plates are coated by dipping into a slurry of silica and then dried, give very variable results and are not recommended. In general, home-made plates tend to give silica layers that are much more fragile than those of commercially available plates and chromatographic performance tends to be much less reproducible. Experience suggests that it is best to use one particular brand of commercially available plates. However, even with commercial plates dramatic batch-to-batch variations in retention and sensitivity to certain spray reagents may still be encountered.

4.4.2 Sample application

Some commercial plates are supplied with special adsorbent layers to simplify application of the sample. Normally, however, the sample is placed directly on to the silica-gel layer. The plate should be prepared by marking the origin with a light pencil line at least 1 cm from the bottom of the plate — care should be taken not to disturb the silica surface in any way. A line should then be scored on the plate 10 cm above the origin to indicate the optimum position of the solvent front; other distances may be used if required. It is advisable when using 20 × 20-cm plates to score columns 2 cm in width vertically up the plate with, say, a pencil since this minimizes edge effects, as discussed in section 4.4.3.

The samples and any standards should be applied carefully at the origin in the appropriate columns, using a micropipette or syringe so as to form spots no more than than 5 mm in diameter. If larger spots are produced, resolution will be impaired when the chromatogram is developed. The volume of solvent applied should be kept to a minimum; typically 5–10 μl of solution containing about 10 μg of analyte. Sample extracts reconstituted as appropriate should be applied first, followed by the standards or mixtures of standards; this sequence minimizes the risk of cross-contamination. Glass capillaries intended for use in melting-point apparatus can easily be drawn out in the flame of a microburner to give disposable micropipettes with a very fine point. Ideally, the solvent used in applying the sample should be the same as that used to develop the chromatogram, but this is not always practicable; methanol will usually prove satisfactory. The plate may be heated with a hair-drier, for example, to increase the speed of evaporation of the spotting solvent, but it must be allowed to cool before development starts and there is a risk of loss of volatile analytes such as amfetamines.

4.4.3 Developing the chromatogram

Glass TLC development tanks are available from many suppliers and normally have a ground-glass rim which forms an airtight seal with a glass cover plate. A small amount of silicone lubricant jelly may be used to secure the seal. Some tanks have a well at the bottom which reduces the amount of solvent required. Most of the procedures in this manual recommend the use of plates and tanks of standard size, but smaller tanks are advantageous if smaller plates are used. All tanks should be lined with filter-paper or blotting paper on three sides and the solvent should be added at least 30 minutes before the chromatogram is to be developed. This helps to produce an atmosphere saturated with solvent vapour, which in turn aids reproducible chromatography. Some TLC mobile phases consist of a single solvent but most are mixtures; possibly the most widely used mobile phase in analytical toxicology is ethyl acetate/methanol/concentrated ammonium hydroxide (EMA; see section 5.2.3). It is important to prepare mobile phases daily, since their composition may change with time because of evaporation or chemical reaction. In particular, loss of ammonia, not only from the mobile phase but also from opened reagent bottles, causes many problems.

The chromatogram is developed by placing the loaded plate in the uniformly saturated tank, ensuring that the level of the solvent is above the bottom edge of the silica layer on the plate but below the level of the spots applied to the plate, and quickly replacing the lid. The chromatogram should be observed to ensure that the solvent front is rising up the plate uniformly. Usually the solvent front will show curvature at the edges of the plate; more serious curvature or bowing may be observed if the tank atmosphere is not sufficiently saturated with solvent vapour. This effect can be minimized by dividing the plate into 2-cm columns as indicated in section 4.4.2. The chromatogram should be allowed to develop for the intended distance, usually 10 cm from the origin. The plate should then be taken from the tank, placed in a fume cupboard or under a fume hood and allowed to dry. This process may be enhanced by blowing warm air (from a hair-drier) over the plate for several minutes until all traces of solvent have been removed. This can be especially important with ammoniacal mobile phases, since the presence of residual ammonia affects the reactions observed with certain spray reagents.

4.4.4 *Visualizing the chromatogram*

When the chromatogram has been developed and the plate dried, the chromatogram should be examined under ultraviolet light (at 254 nm and 366 nm) and the positions of any fluorescent compounds (spots) noted. This stage is essential if a fluorescent marker has been added to the silica, as any compounds present appear as dark areas against a fluorescent background. However, in analytical toxicology the use of chromagenic chemical detection reagents generally gives more useful information, as discussed in section 5.2.3, and in the appropriate monographs (section 6). Plates can be dipped in reagent but, unless special precautions are taken, the structure of the silica tends to be lost and the chromatogram destroyed. Thus, the reagent is normally lightly applied as an aerosol, using a commercial spray bottle attached to a compressed air or nitrogen line. Varying the line pressure varies the density of the aerosol and thus the amount of reagent reaching the chromatogram in a given time.

Normally, the plate should be sprayed in an inverted position, since this avoids the risk of excess reagent being drawn up the plate by capillary action and destroying the lower part of the chromatogram. Glass plates can be used to mask portions of the plate if columns are to be sprayed with different reagents. Alternatively, if plastic or aluminium plates are used then columns can be cut up and sprayed separately. The appearance of certain compounds may change with time, and it is important to record results as quickly and carefully as possible, noting any changes with time. A standardized recording system is valuable for reference purposes, as discussed in section 5.2.3. Many spray reagents are extremely toxic — **always** use a fume cupboard or hood when spraying TLC plates.

4.4.5 *Retention factors*

TLC results are usually recorded as retention factors. The retention factor (R_f) is defined as follows:

$$R_f = \frac{\text{Distance travelled from the origin by the analyte}}{\text{Distance travelled from the origin by the solvent front}}$$

A more convenient value is $R_f \times 100$ (hR_f), especially if a standard length of chromatogram of 10 cm is always used, since then hR_f is equal to the distance in millimetres travelled from the origin by the analyte.

There are many factors that influence the reproducibility of hR_f values including (1) the TLC plate itself, (2) the amount of analyte applied to the plate, (3) the development distance, (4) the degree of tank saturation, and (5) the ambient temperature. However, the influence of these factors can be minimized if standard (reference) compounds are analysed together with each sample. For unknown substances, it is a relatively simple procedure to obtain a corrected hR_f value from a calibration graph constructed from experimentally observed values of sample and reference compounds. However, a further complicating factor is that the chromatography of compounds that originate from biological extracts may be different from that of the pure substances because of interferences from additional material present in sample extracts (matrix effects) (see section 5.2.3).

4.5 Ultraviolet and visible spectrophotometry

A number of the quantitative methods described in the monographs (section 6) employ ultraviolet (UV) (200–400 nm) or visible (400–800 nm) spectrophotometry. The major problem encountered with this technique is interference, and some form of sample purification, such as solvent extraction or microdiffusion (see section 4.3), is usually employed. The spectrophotometer may be of the single-beam or double-beam type. With a single-beam instrument, light passes from the source through a monochromator and then via a sample cell to the detector. With double-beam instruments, light from the monochromator passes through a beam-splitting device and then via separate sample and reference cells to the detector. Double-beam instruments with auto-mated wavelength scanning and a variety of other features are also available.

4.5.1 The Beer-Lambert law

In spectrophotometry, the relationship between the intensity of light entering and leaving a cell is governed by the Beer-Lambert law, which states that, for a solution with an absorbing solute in a transparent solvent, the fraction of the incident light absorbed is proportional to the number of solute molecules in the light path, i.e.,

$$\log_{10} I_0/I = kcb$$

where
I_0 is the incident light intensity,
I is the transmitted light intensity,
c is the solute concentration (g/l),
b is the path length (cm),
k is the absorptivity of the system.

The constant k is a fundamental property of the solute, but also depends on temperature, wavelength and solvent. The term $\log_{10} I_0 / I$ is known as absorbance (A) and, for dilute solutions only, is linearly related to both solute concentration and path length. In older textbooks it was known as optical density (OD) or extinction coefficient (E), but these terms are now obsolete. The specific absorbance ($A_{1\%}$, 1 cm) is the absorbance of a 1% (w/v) (10 g/litre) solution of the solute in a cell of 1-cm path length, and is usually written in the shortened form A_1^1.

31

4.5.2. *Spectrophotometric assays*

With all types of spectrophotometer it is important to ensure that the monochromator is correctly aligned. This can be checked by observing the absorbance maxima (λ_{max}) of a known reference solution or material. For example, a holmium oxide glass filter has major peaks at a number of important wavelengths (241.5 nm, 279.4 nm, 287.5 nm, 333.7 nm, 360.9 nm, 418.4 nm, 453.2 nm, 536.2 nm and 637.5 nm). A simple method of checking the photometric accuracy is to measure the absorbance of an acidic potassium dichromate solution (see Table 10).

It is important that the cells used in the spectrophotometer are of the correct specification and that they are scrupulously clean. Glass and certain types of plastic cells are suitable for measurements in the visible region (> 400 nm), but only fused silica or quartz cells should be used for UV work (< 400 nm). Normally, cells of 1-cm path length are used, but cells of 2-cm or 4-cm path length can sometimes enhance sensitivity.

Double-beam spectrophotometers have the advantage that background absorbance from reagents, solvents, etc., can be allowed for by including a blank (analyte-free) extract in the reference position. Normally, an extract of blank plasma or serum is used in the reference cell, but purified water can be used in certain assays. In high sensitivity work, it is important to use matching cells, i.e., cells with similar absorbance values, for the test and reference measurements. Pairs of matched cells can be purchased and should be kept together.

As mentioned previously, a major worry in many spectrophotometric assays is the risk of interference from co-ingested drugs or other compounds. However, some information as to the purity of a sample extract can often be obtained by examining the UV absorption spectrum. While this can be done most easily using an instrument with a

Table 10. Photometric calibration using potassium dichromate (60.00 mg/l) in aqueous sulfuric acid (0.005 mol/l)[a]

Wavelength (nm)	Specific absorbance (A_1^1)
235	124.5
257	144.0
313	48.6
350	106.6

[a] Values from *British Pharmacopoeia*, London, Her Majesty's Stationery Office, 1980.

built-in scanning facility, it can also be performed manually on simpler instruments. UV spectra of extracts of stomach contents or scene residues can also give useful qualitative information, and can be used as an adjunct to the drug screening procedure described in section 5.2. However, such an approach is only practical with an instrument with a built-in scanning facility.[a]

---

[a] UV absorption spectra of many compounds of interest are given in *Clarke's isolation and identification of drugs* (Moffat, 1986) (see Bibliography, section 1), but again care is needed to ensure that the pH/solvent combination employed is the same as that used to produce the reference spectrum.

5

Qualitative tests for poisons

Many difficulties may be encountered when performing qualitative tests for poisons, especially if laboratory facilities are limited. The poisons may include gases, such as carbon monoxide, drugs, solvents, pesticides, metal salts, corrosive liquids (acids, alkalis) and natural toxins. Some poisons may be pure chemicals and others complex natural products. Not surprisingly, there is no comprehensive range of tests for all poisons in all samples.

When certain compounds are suggested by the history or clinical findings, simple tests may be performed using the procedures given in the monographs (section 6). However, in the absence of clinical or other evidence to indicate the poison(s) involved, a defined series of tests (a screen) is needed. It is usually advisable to perform this series of tests routinely, since circumstantial evidence of poisoning is often misleading. Similarly, the analysis should not end after the first positive result, since additional unsuspected compounds may be present.

The sequence of analyses outlined in section 5.2 will detect and identify a number of poisons in commonly available specimens (urine, stomach contents, and scene residues, i.e., material such as tablets or suspect solutions found with or near to the patient) using a minimum of apparatus and reagents. The compounds detected include many that give rise to nonspecific features, such as drowsiness, coma or convulsions, and which will not be indicated by clinical examination alone. Poisons for which specific therapy is available, such as acetylsalicylic acid and paracetamol, are also included. The analysis takes about 2 hours and may be modified to incorporate common local poisons if appropriate tests are available.

5.1 Collection, storage and use of specimens

5.1.1 Clinical liaison

Good liaison between the clinician and the analyst is of vital importance if the results of a toxicological analysis are to be useful (see section 2). Ideally, this liaison should commence before the specimens are collected, and any special sample requirements for particular analytes noted. At the very least, a request form should be completed to accompany the

34

specimens to the laboratory. An example of such a form is given in Fig. 2.

Before starting an analysis it is important to obtain as much information about the patient as possible (medical, social and occupational history, treatment given, and the results of laboratory or other investigations), as discussed in sections 2 and 3. It is also important to be aware of the time that elapsed between ingestion or exposure and the collection of samples, since this may influence the interpretation of results. All relevant information about a patient gathered in conversation

Fig. 2. Example of an analytical toxicology request form

ANALYTICAL TOXICOLOGY REQUEST To: [Insert laboratory name, address and telephone no.] Discuss special requirements BEFORE sending samples.	Date/time of admission:
	Date/time of ingestion or exposure:
	Drugs prescribed or used in treatment:
Doctor (PLEASE PRINT): Telephone/bleep no: Hospital address for report: Signed: Date:	Drugs/poisons claimed or suspected:
Patient: Other names: Age/date of birth: Sex: Consultant: Ward: Reference no:	Clinical details/investigation required/priority:

Sample type	Date	Time
Blood (10 ml heparinized)		
Urine (50 ml; catheter yes/no)		
Stomach contents (50 ml)		
Other (give details)		

with the clinician, nurse, or poisons information service should be recorded in the laboratory using the external request form (Fig. 2) or a suitably modified version of this form.

5.1.2 *Specimen transport and storage*

Specimens sent for analysis must be clearly labelled with the patient's full name, the date and time of collection, and the nature of the specimen if this is not self-evident. This is especially important if large numbers of patients have been involved in a particular incident, or a number of specimens have been obtained from one patient. Confusion frequently arises when one or more blood samples are separated in a local laboratory and the original containers are discarded. When the plasma/serum samples are forwarded subsequently to the toxicology laboratory for analysis, it can be difficult, if not impossible, to ascertain which is which.

The date and time of receipt of all specimens by the laboratory should be recorded and a unique identifying number assigned to each specimen (see section 4.1.6). Containers of volatile materials, such as organic solvents, should be packaged separately from biological specimens to avoid the possibility of cross-contamination. All biological specimens should be stored at 4 °C prior to analysis, if possible, and ideally any specimen remaining after the analysis should be kept at 4 °C for 3–4 weeks in case further analyses are required. In view of the medicolegal implications of some poison cases (for example, if it is not clear how the poison was administered or if the patient dies) then any specimen remaining should be kept (preferably at −20 °C) until investigation of the incident has been concluded.

5.1.3 *Urine*

Urine is useful for screening tests as it is often available in large volumes and usually contains higher concentrations of drugs or other poisons than blood. The presence of metabolites may sometimes assist identification if chromatographic techniques are used. A 50-ml specimen from an adult, collected in a sealed, sterile container, is sufficient for most purposes; no preservative should be added. The sample should be obtained as soon as possible, ideally before any drug therapy is initiated. However, drugs such as tricyclic antidepressants (amitriptyline, imipramine) cause urinary retention, and thus a very early specimen may contain insignificant amounts of poison. Conversely, little poison may remain in specimens taken many hours or days later, even though the patient may be very ill, as in acute paracetamol poisoning. If the specimen is obtained by catheterization there is a possibility of contamination with lidocaine. If syrup of ipecacuanha has been given in an unsuccessful attempt to induce emesis there is a possibility of emetine being present in the urine.

5.1.4 *Stomach contents*

Stomach contents may include vomit, gastric aspirate and stomach washings — it is important to obtain the first sample of washings, since later samples may be very dilute. A volume of at least 20 ml is required to carry out a wide range of tests; no preservative should be added. This can be a very variable sample and additional procedures such as homogenization followed by filtration and/or centrifugation may be required to produce a fluid amenable to analysis. However, it is the best sample on which to perform certain tests. If obtained soon after ingestion, large amounts of poison may be present while metabolites, which may complicate some tests, are usually absent. An immediate clue to certain compounds may be given by the smell; it may be possible to identify tablets or capsules simply by inspection. Note that emetine from syrup of ipecacuanha may be present, especially in children (section 2.2.1).

5.1.5 *Scene residues*

It is important that all bottles or other containers and other suspect materials found with or near the patient (scene residues) are retained for analysis if necessary since they may be related to the poisoning episode. There is always the possibility that the original contents of containers have been discarded and replaced either with innocuous material or with more noxious ingredients such as acid, bleach or pesticides. Note that it is always best to analyse biological specimens in the first instance if possible.

A few milligrams of scene residues are usually sufficient for the tests described here. Dissolve solid material in a few millilitres of water or other appropriate solvent. Use as small an amount as possible in each test, in order to conserve sufficient for possible further tests.

5.1.6 *Blood*

Blood (plasma or serum) is normally reserved for quantitative assays but for some poisons, such as carbon monoxide and cyanide, whole blood has to be used for qualitative tests. For adults, a 10-ml sample should be collected in a heparinized tube on admission. In addition, a 2-ml sample should be collected in a fluoride/oxalate tube, if ethanol poisoning is suspected. Note that tubes of this type available commercially contain the equivalent of about 1 g/l fluoride, whereas about 10 g/l fluoride (40 mg sodium fluoride per 2 ml of blood) is needed to inhibit fully microbial action in such specimens. The use of disinfectant swabs containing alcohols (ethanol, propan-2-ol) should be avoided. The sample should be dispensed with care: the vigorous discharge of blood though a syringe needle can cause sufficient haemolysis to invalidate a serum iron or potassium assay.

In general, there are no significant differences in the concentrations of poisons between plasma and serum. However, if a compound is not present to any extent within erythrocytes, the use of lysed whole blood will result in considerable dilution of the specimen. On the other hand, some poisons, such as carbon monoxide, cyanide and lead, are found primarily in erythrocytes and thus whole blood is needed for such measurements. A heparinized whole blood sample will give either whole blood or plasma as appropriate. The space above the blood in the tube (headspace) should be minimized if carbon monoxide poisoning is suspected.

5.2 Analysis of urine, stomach contents and scene residues

If any tests are to influence immediate clinical management, the results must be available within 2–3 hours of receipt of the specimen. Of course, a positive result does not in itself confirm poisoning, since such a result may arise from incidental or occupational exposure to the poison in question or the use of drugs in treatment. In some cases, the presence of more than one poison may complicate the analysis, and examination of further specimens from the patient may be required. A quantitative analysis carried out on whole blood or plasma may be needed to confirm poisoning, but this may not be possible if laboratory facilities are limited. It is important to discuss the scope and limitations of the tests performed with the clinician concerned, and to maintain high standards of laboratory practice (see section 4.1), especially when performing tests on an emergency basis. It may be better to offer no result rather than misleading data based on an unreliable test. In any event, it is valuable to have a worksheet to record the analytical results. An example of such a sheet is given in Fig. 3.

The qualitative scheme given below, possibly modified to suit local needs, should be followed in every case unless there are good reasons (such as insufficient sample) for omitting part of the screen, since this will

Fig. 3. Example of an analytical toxicology worksheet

TOXICOLOGY WORKSHEET					
Patient:	Doctor:				
Hospital:	Telephone/bleep no:				
Assay requested:	Priority:				

Sample type	Laboratory no.	Date	Time	Laboratory no.	Test performed
					Qualitative analysis
					1. Salicylates
					2. Phenothiazines
					3. Imipramine
					4. Trichloro compounds
					5. Paracetamol
					6. Paraquat/diquat
					7. Ethanol
					8. Chlorates, etc.
					9. Iron
					10. TLC acidic + basic drugs

Substance	Laboratory no.	Concentration			
		11.			
		12.			
		13.			
		14.			
		15.			
		16.			
		17.			
		Analyst:			Date/Time:

39

Table 11. Some compounds not detected in urine by the drug screening procedure

Group	Compound
Inorganic ions	arsenic, barium, bismuth, borate, bromide, cadmium, copper, cyanide, fluoride, lead, lithium, mercury, sulfide, thallium
Organic chemicals	camphor, carbon disulfide, carbon monoxide, carbon tetrachloride, dichloromethane, ethylene glycol, formates, oxalates, petroleum distillates, phenols, tetrachloroethylene, toluene, 1,1,1-trichloroethane
Drugs	benzodiazepines, coumarin anticoagulants, dapsone, digoxin, ethchlorvynol, glyceryl trinitrate, meprobamate, monoamine oxidase inhibitors, theophylline, tolbutamide
Pesticides	carbamate pesticides, chloralose, chlorophenoxy herbicides, dinitrophenol pesticides, fluoroacetates, hydroxybenzonitrile herbicides, methyl bromide, organochlorine pesticides, organophosphorus pesticides, pentachlorophenol

provide a good chance of detecting any poisons present. The scheme has three parts: physical examination, colour tests and thin-layer chromatography, and is designed primarily for the analysis of urine samples. However, most of the tests and some additional ones are also applicable, with due precautions, to stomach contents and scene residues. Some compounds and groups of compounds not normally detected using this procedure are listed in Table 11. Simple tests for many of these compounds are given in the monographs (section 6).

5.2.1 *Physical examination of the specimen*

Urine

High concentrations of some drugs or metabolites can impart characteristic colours to urine (Table 12). Deferoxamine or methylene blue given in treatment may colour urine red or blue, respectively. Strong-smelling poisons such as camphor, ethchlorvynol and methyl salicylate can sometimes be recognized in urine since they are excreted in part unchanged. Acetone may arise from metabolism of propan-2-ol. Turbidity may be due to underlying pathology (blood, microorganisms, casts, epithelial cells), or to carbonates, phosphates or urates in amorphous or microcrystalline forms. Such findings should not be ignored,

Table 12. Some possible causes of coloured urine

Colour	Possible cause
Brown or black (intensifying on standing)	nitrobenzene, phenols, rhubarb (liver failure)
Yellow or orange	cascara, fluorescein, phenolphthalein, nitrofurantoin, senna
Wine red or brown	aloin, phenothiazines, phenytoin, phenol-phthalein, quinine, warfarin (haematuria)
Blue or green	amitriptyline, indometacin, phenols

even though they may not be related to the poisoning. Chronic therapy with sulfonamides may give rise to yellow or greenish brown crystals in neutral or alkaline urine. Phenytoin, primidone, and sultiame form crystals in urine following overdosage, while characteristic colourless crystals of calcium oxalate form at neutral pH after ingestion of ethylene glycol (Fig. 4).

Fig. 4. Calcium oxalate crystals, as found in urine by microscopy after ingestion of ethylene glycol

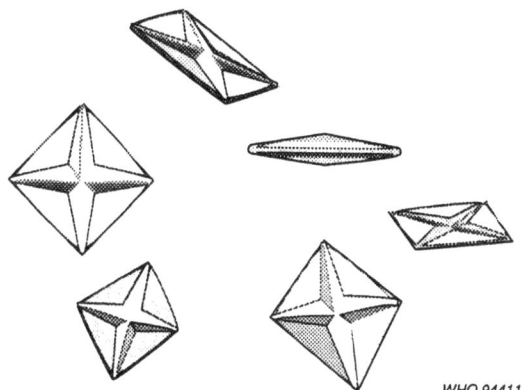

WHO 94411

Stomach contents and scene residues

Some characteristic smells associated with particular substances are listed in Table 13. Many other compounds (for example, ethchlorvynol, methyl salicylate, paraldehyde, phenelzine) also have distinctive smells. Very low or very high pH may indicate ingestion of acid or alkali, while a green/blue colour suggests the presence of iron or copper salts. Microscopic examination using a polarizing microscope may reveal the presence of tablet or capsule debris. Starch granules used as a filler in

Table 13. Characteristic smells associated with particular poisons[a]

Smell	Possible cause
Bitter almonds	cyanide
Fruity	alcohols (including ethanol), esters
Garlic	arsenic, phosphorus
Mothballs	camphor
Pears	chloral
Petrol	petroleum distillates (may be vehicle in pesticide formulation)
Phenolic	disinfectants, phenols
Stale tobacco	nicotine
Shoe polish	nitrobenzene
Sweet	chloroform and other halogenated hydrocarbons

[a] **Take care**: specimens containing cyanide may give off hydrogen cyanide, especially if acidified — not everyone can detect hydrogen cyanide by smell. Similarly sulfides evolve hydrogen sulfide — the ability to detect hydrogen sulfide (rotten egg smell) is lost at higher concentrations.

Some tablets and capsules are best identified using crossed polarizing filters, when they appear as bright grains marked with a dark Maltese cross.

Undegraded tablets or capsules and any plant remains or specimens of plants thought to have been ingested should be examined separately. The local poisons information service will normally have access to publications or other aids to the identification of tablets or capsules by weight, markings, colour, shape and possibly other physical features.

5.2.2 Colour tests

The nine qualitative tests described here are based on simple colour reactions and cover a number of important drugs and other poisons. Full descriptions of these tests are given in the respective monographs (section 6), together with details of common sources of interference and detection limits. Other tests, such as the Reinsch test for antimony, arsenic, bismuth and mercury, are not discussed further here, but full details are given in the respective monographs.

Of the tests outlined (Table 14), that for salicylates such as acetylsalicylic acid (aspirin) (Trinder's test, also known as the ferric chloride test) is best performed on urine rather than stomach contents or scene residues, since acetylsalicylic acid itself does not react unless hydrolysed. Most of the others may be performed using either specimen, but the tests for

Table 14. Recommended qualitative colour tests

1. Salicylic acid (including acetylsalicylic acid (aspirin)) — Trinder's test

Add 100 μl of Trinder's reagent (a mixture of 40 g of mercuric chloride in 850 ml of water and 120 ml of aqueous hydrochloric acid (1 mol/l) and 40 g of hydrated ferric nitrate, diluted to 1 l with water) to 2 ml of urine and mix for 5 seconds. A violet colour indicates the presence of salicylates.

If only stomach contents or scene residues are available, hydrolyse by heating with 0.5 mol/l hydrochloric acid on a boiling water-bath for 2 minutes, and neutralize with 0.5 mol/l sodium hydroxide before performing the test (see section 6.99).

If a positive result is obtained in this test, carry out a quantitative assay on plasma/serum (see section 6.99).

2. Phenothiazines — FPN test

Add 1 ml of FPN reagent (a mixture of 5 ml of aqueous ferric chloride solution (50 g/litre), 45 ml of aqueous perchloric acid (200 g/kg) and 50 ml of aqueous nitric acid (500 ml/litre)) to 1 ml of sample and mix for 5 seconds. Colours ranging from pink to red, orange, violet or blue suggest the presence of phenothiazines.

Positive results should be confirmed by thin-layer chromatography (section 5.2.3).

3. Imipramine and related compounds — Forrest test

Add 1 ml of Forrest reagent (a mixture of 25 ml of aqueous potassium dichromate (2 g/l), 25 ml of aqueous sulfuric acid (300 ml/l), 25 ml of aqueous perchloric acid (200 g/kg) and 25 ml of aqueous nitric acid (500 ml/l)) to 0.5 ml of sample and mix for 5 seconds. A yellow-green colour deepening through dark green to blue indicates the presence of imipramine or related compounds.

Positive results should be confirmed by thin-layer chromatography (section 5.2.3).

4. Trichloro compounds (including chloral hydrate, chloroform, dichloralphenazone and trichloroethylene) — Fujiwara test

To three 10-ml tubes, add respectively 1-ml portions of (*a*) sample, (*b*) purified water (blank test — **essential**), and (*c*) aqueous trichloroacetic acid (10 mg/l). Add 1 ml of sodium hydroxide solution (5 mol/l) and 1 ml of pyridine to each tube, mix carefully and heat in a boiling water-bath for 2 minutes. An intense red/purple colour in the top (pyridine) layer of tube (*a*) (as in tube (*c*)) indicates the presence of trichloro compounds; tube (*b*) should show no coloration.

5. Paracetamol, phenacetin — *o*-cresol/ammonia test

Add 0.5 ml of concentrated hydrochloric acid to 0.5 ml of sample, heat in a boiling water-bath for 10 minutes and cool. Add 1 ml of aqueous *o*-cresol solution (10 g/l) to 0.2 ml of the hydrolysate, add 2 ml of ammonium hydroxide solution (4 mol/l), and mix for 5 seconds. A strong blue to blue-black colour, which forms immediately, indicates the presence of paracetamol or phenacetin.

Table 14 (contd.)

If a positive result is obtained in this test carry out a quantitative assay for paracetamol on plasma or serum (see section 6.83).

6. Paraquat, diquat — dithionite test

Add 0.5 ml of aqueous ammonium hydroxide (2 mol/l) to 1 ml of test solution, mix for 5 seconds and add about 20 mg of solid sodium dithionite. A strong, blue to blue-black colour indicates paraquat; diquat gives a yellow-green colour, but this is insignificant in the presence of paraquat.

If the colour fades on continued agitation in air and is restored by adding further sodium dithionite, paraquat or diquat is confirmed.

7. Ethanol and other volatile reducing agents — dichromate test

Apply 50 μl of potassium dichromate (25 g/l in aqueous sulfuric acid (500 ml/l)) to a strip of glass-fibre filter-paper and insert the paper in the neck of a test-tube containing 1 ml of urine. Lightly stopper the tube and place in a boiling water-bath for 2 minutes. A change in colour from orange to green indicates the presence of volatile reducing substances.

If a positive result is obtained in this test carry out a quantitative assay for ethanol on blood (see section 6.46).

8. Chlorates and other oxidizing agents — diphenylamine test[a]

Carefully add 0.5 ml of diphenylamine (10 g/l in concentrated sulfuric acid) to 0.5 ml of filtered stomach contents or scene residue. A strong blue colour which develops rapidly indicates the presence of oxidizing agents.

9. Ferrous and ferric iron — ferricyanide/ferrocyanide test[a]

To 50 μl of filtered stomach contents or scene residue add 100 μl of aqueous hydrochloric acid (2 mol/l) and 50 μl of aqueous potassium ferricyanide solution (10 g/l). To a further 50 μl of sample add 100 μl of hydrochloric acid and 50 μl of potassium ferrocyanide solution (10 g/l). A deep blue precipitate with potassium ferricyanide or ferrocyanide indicates the presence of ferrous or ferric iron.

If a positive result is obtained in this test carry out a quantitative assay for iron on serum (see section 6.61).

---

[a] Tests for use on stomach contents or scene residues only.

chlorates and other oxidizing agents and for ferrous or ferric iron can only be carried out on stomach contents or scene residues. Examples of the colours obtained in these tests are given in Plates 1–8.

5.2.3 *Thin-layer chromatography*

The aim of the scheme outlined below is to obtain as much information as possible in a short time and with a minimum of sample. Drugs and, in some cases, metabolites present are extracted from the sample into an organic solvent under acidic and alkaline conditions. The extracts are analysed by thin-layer chromatography (TLC) on one plate using a single solvent system. The basic extract is acidified during the evaporation stage to minimize loss of volatile bases such as amfetamines. If the sample volume is limited, the acidic and basic extractions can be performed sequentially on the same portion of the specimen. However, it is important that the pH change between extractions is accomplished satisfactorily. Extracts of stomach contents may contain fatty material, which makes chromatographic analysis difficult, and purification by re-extraction into aqueous acid or alkali may be required.

Although simple examination of the developed chromatogram under ultraviolet light (254 nm and 366 nm) may reveal the presence of fluorescent compounds such as quinine, the use of a number of spray (visualization) reagents widens the scope of the analysis and increases the confidence of any identifications.

The recommended TLC visualization reagents are as follows:

1. Mercurous nitrate reagent (acidic extract), which gives white spots with a grey centre on a darker background with barbiturates and related compounds such as glutethimide.
2. Acidified iodoplatinate reagent (basic extract), which gives mainly purple, blue or brown spots with a range of basic and neutral drugs and metabolites. Note that some authors recommend neutral iodoplatinate, which is more stable and which gives similar reactions with many basic drugs; this is oversprayed with sulfuric acid (500 ml/l) which facilitates reactions with neutral compounds such as caffeine and phenazone (from dichloralphenazone) .
3. Mandelin's reagent (basic extract) gives colours ranging from blue and green to orange and red with a variety of basic compounds. Some, especially tricyclic antidepressants such as amitriptyline and nortriptyline, give fluorescent spots if viewed under ultraviolet light (366 nm) after spraying with this reagent.
4. Sulfuric acid (500 ml/l) (basic extract) alone gives red, purple or blue spots with many phenothiazines and their metabolites. This is especially valuable since some phenothiazines (chlorpromazine, for example) are given therapeutically in relatively high doses and have many metabolites, which can give a very confusing picture if unrecognized.

Of course, many additional mobile phase and spray reagent combinations could be used as well as, or in place of, those suggested here, and details of some are given in the references listed in the Bibliography (p. 234) and in the monographs (section 6). For example,

Table 15. Thin-layer chromatography hR$_f$ values (eluent EMA) and colour reactions (rim colour) with spray reagents

Compound	hR$_f$	Visualization reagent				
		Mercurous nitrate	Acidified iodo-platinate	Mandelin's reagent (visible light)[a]	Mandelin's reagent (UV 366 nm)[a]	Sulfuric acid (500 ml/l)
3-acetylmorphine	24	—	blue	—	—	—
6-acetylmorphine (diamorphine metabolites)	48	—	blue	—	—	—
N-acetylprocainamide (procainamide metabolite)	—	—	blue	—	—	—
amfetamine	44	—	blue	—	—	—
aminophenazone	61	—	blue	—	—	—
amiodarone	82	—	blue	—	—	—
amitriptyline	70	—	blue	pale blue	blue (yellow)	—
amobarbital	40	white-grey	—	—	—	—
atropine	25	—	blue	—	—	—
barbital	33	white-grey	—	—	—	—
benzoctamine	77	—	purple	grey	—	—
benzoylecgonine (cocaine metabolite)	2	—	blue	—	—	—
brallobarbital	29	white-grey	—	—	—	—
brucine	26	—	blue	—	—	—
butobarbital	39	white-grey	—	—	—	—
caffeine	50	—	blue	—	—	—
carbamazepine	57	—	blue	pale blue	green	—
chloroquine	52	—	blue	—	pale blue	—
chlorpromazine	70	—	purple	red	—	red

			purple	pink	orange (yellow)	pink
chlorprothixene	74	—	purple	—	—	—
clomethiazole	74	—	blue	—	pale blue	—
clomipramine	72	—	purple	green-blue	—	—
cocaine	77	—	purple	—	—	—
codeine	35	—	black	pale blue	—	—
cotinine (nicotine metabolite)	40	—	blue	—	—	—
cyclizine	68	—	blue	yellow	—	—
cyclobarbital	35	white-grey	—	—	—	—
desipramine	41	—	purple	dark blue	—	—
dextropropoxyphene	80	—	purple	grey	blue (brown)	—
diamorphine (heroin)^b	51	—	blue	pale blue	—	—
dibenzepin	57	—	purple	pale blue	yellow	—
dihydrocodeine	27	—	black	pale blue	—	—
diphenhydramine	68	—	blue	yellow	yellow	—
dosulepin	65	—	purple	pale blue	pale blue	—
doxepin	65	—	purple	brown	orange	—
emetine	62	—	purple	white	—	—
ephedrine	27	—	blue	—	—	—
ethylmorphine	36	—	blue	—	—	—
fenfluramine	60	—	blue	—	—	—
glutethimide	78	white-grey	—	—	—	—
haloperidol	74	—	purple	—	—	—
hexobarbital	51	white-grey	—	—	—	—
imipramine	67	—	purple	dark blue	pale blue	—
iproniazid	42	—	blue	violet	—	—
isoniazid	29	—	blue	—	—	—
levorphanol	41	—	brown	white	—	—
lidocaine	80	—	blue	—	—	—
maprotiline	35	—	blue	blue	—	—

47

Basic analytical toxicology

Table 15 (contd.)

Compound	hR$_f$	Visualization reagent				
		Mercurous nitrate	Acidified iodo-platinate	Mandelin's reagent (visible light)[a]	Mandelin's reagent (UV 366 nm)[a]	Sulfuric acid (500 ml/l)
mefenamic acid	14	—	—	blue-grey	—	—
metamfetamine	35	—	blue	—	—	—
methadone	77	—	brown	white	—	—
methaqualone	78	—	—	—	green	—
methylephedrine	35	—	blue	—	—	—
methyprylon	63	white-grey	—	—	—	—
metixene	70	—	purple	blue	purple	—
morphine	20	—	blue	—	—	—
nicotine	61	—	blue	—	—	—
norephedrine (ephedrine metabolite)	28	—	blue	—	—	—
norpethidine (pethidine metabolite)	34	—	purple	—	—	—
nortriptyline (amitriptyline metabolite)	45	—	blue	pale blue	blue (yellow)	—
opipramol	38	—	blue	yellow	pale green	—
orphenadrine	70	—	blue	yellow	pale blue	—
oxycodone	60	—	purple	white	purple	—
pentazocine	72	—	brown	grey	pale blue	—
perphenazine	43	—	—	red	—	red
pethidine	62	—	purple	—	—	—
phenazone (from dichloralphenazone)	44	—	blue	—	—	—

phenelzine	83	—	—	pink	—	—
phenobarbital	29	white-grey	—	—	—	—
phenytoin	39	white-grey	—	—	—	—
primidone	40	white-grey	—	—	—	—
procainamide	39	—	blue	red	—	red
prochlorperazine	54	—	blue	red-brown	—	red
promazine	65	—	—	red	—	red
promethazine	65	—	purple	blue	purple	—
propranolol	52	—	blue	—	—	—
protriptyline	41	—	blue	orange (purple)	brown (green)	—
quinidine	52	—	purple	—	blue	—
quinine	52	—	purple	—	blue	—
secobarbital	42	white-grey	—	—	—	—
strychnine	33	—	blue	—	—	—
theophylline	10	white-grey	—	—	—	—
thiopental	49	white-grey	—	—	—	—
thioridazine	67	—	purple-brown	blue-green	blue	purple
tofenacin (orphenadrine metabolite)	—	—	blue	yellow	pale blue	—
tolbutamide	12	—	blue	—	—	—
tranylcypromine	60	—	—	violet	—	—
trazodone	68	—	purple	purple	blue	—
trimipramine	80	—	blue	dark blue	—	—
trifluoperazine	56	—	purple	pink	—	pink
verapamil	74	—	blue	—	—	—

[a] With certain compounds, there may be a colour difference between the centre and the outer part of the spot; this is indicated by the mention of a second colour in parentheses.

[b] Diamorphine itself is not found in urine, but is detected as monoacetyl morphine and morphine conjugates.

49

methanol:concentrated ammonium hydroxide (99:1.5) (methanol:ammonia, MA) is widely used in the analysis of basic drugs, and is especially useful in the detection of morphine and related opioids (see section 6.73). Of the spray reagents, Marquis' reagent gives a variety of colours with different basic drugs, and is again especially valuable for the detection of morphine and other opioids which give blue/violet colours.

In all cases, the colour obtained from a particular compound may vary depending on concentration, the presence of co-eluting compounds, the duration and intensity of spraying, and the type of silica used in the manufacture of the plate, among other factors. Some compounds may show a gradation or even a change in colour from the edge of the spot towards the centre (usually a concentration effect), while the intensity or even the nature of the colour obtained may vary with time. A further problem is that the interpretation and recording of colour reactions are very subjective. It is thus important to analyse authentic compounds, ideally on the same plate as the sample extracts. Even so, compounds present in sample extracts sometimes show slightly different chromatograms from the pure compounds owing to the presence of co-extracted material. Interfering neutral compounds, especially fatty acids from stomach contents, can be removed by back-extraction of acidic or basic compounds into dilute base or acid, respectively (the neutral compounds stay in the organic extract), followed by re-extraction into organic solvent.

Detailed records of each analysis should be kept, not only for medicolegal purposes, but also to establish a reference data bank to aid in the interpretation of results. This can be used to supplement the data given in Table 15 and elsewhere, and has the advantage of being generated in the laboratory actually involved in analysing the specimens.

The recommended TLC screening system is as follows.

Qualitative analysis

Applicable to urine, stomach contents or scene residues.

Reagents and equipment

1. Aqueous hydrochloric acid (1 mol/l).
2. Aqueous sodium hydroxide (0.5 mol/l).
3. Ammonium chloride buffer. Saturated aqueous ammonium chloride adjusted to pH 9 with concentrated ammonium hydroxide (relative density 0.88).
4. Hydrochloric acid (2 ml/l in methanol).
5. Ethyl acetate:methanol:concentrated ammonium hydroxide (EMA) (85:10:5) (relative density 0.88).

6. Mercurous nitrate reagent. Place 1 g of mercurous nitrate in 100 ml of purified water and add concentrated nitric acid (relative density 1.42) until the solution is clear.
7. Acidified iodoplatinate reagent. Mix 0.25 g of platinic chloride, 5 g of potassium iodide and 5 ml of concentrated hydrochloric acid (relative density 1.18) in 100 ml of purified water.
8. Mandelin's reagent. Suspend 1 g of finely powdered ammonium vanadate in 100 ml of concentrated sulfuric acid (relative density 1.86). **Shake well before use.**
9. Aqueous sulfuric acid (500 ml/l).
10. Silica gel thin-layer chromatography plate (20 × 20 cm, 20 μm average particle size; see section 4.4.1).

Standards

All 1 g/l in chloroform:

1. Acidic drugs mixture (amobarbital, mefenamic acid, phenobarbital, theophylline).
2. Basic drugs mixture (amitriptyline, codeine, nicotine, nortriptyline).
3. Phenothiazine mixture (perphenazine, trifluoperazine, thioridazine).

Methods

1. Acidic extract (extract A)
   (a) To 10 ml of urine in a 30-ml glass centrifuge tube add 1 ml of dilute hydrochloric acid and 10 ml of chloroform.
   (b) Shake on a mechanical shaker for 5 minutes, centrifuge in a bench centrifuge for 10 minutes and transfer the lower, organic layer to a 15-ml tapered glass tube.
   (c) Evaporate the extract to dryness on a water-bath at 60 °C under a stream of compressed air.

2. Basic extract (extract B)
   (a) To a further 10 ml of urine in a 30-ml glass tube, add 2 ml of ammonium chloride buffer and 10 ml of chloroform:propan-2-ol (9:1).
   (b) Shake on a mechanical shaker for 5 minutes, centrifuge in a bench centrifuge for 10 minutes and transfer the lower, organic layer to a 15-ml tapered glass tube.
   (c) Add 0.5 ml of methanolic hydrochloric acid (to minimize losses of volatile bases; see section 6.1) and evaporate the extract to dryness in a water-bath at 60 °C under a stream of compressed air.

51

3. Purification of extracts of stomach contents
   (a) Prior to the solvent evaporation stage, add 5 ml of aqueous sodium hydroxide solution to extract A, and 5 ml of aqueous hydrochloric acid to extract B.
   (b) Shake on a mechanical shaker for 5 minutes, centrifuge in a bench centrifuge for 10 minutes and discard both organic layers.
   (c) Add 5 ml of aqueous hydrochloric acid to the aqueous residue from extract A, and 5 ml of ammonium chloride buffer to the aqueous residue from extract B, and re-extract into chloroform or chloroform:propan-2-ol as in methods 1 and 2 above.

Thin-layer chromatography

1. Divide the plate into eight columns by scoring with a pencil (see section 4.4.2). Lightly draw a pencil line about 1 cm from the bottom of the plate to indicate the origin, and score a horizontal line 10 cm from the origin to indicate the limit of development, as shown in Fig. 5.
2. Reconstitute each extract in 100 µl of chloroform:propan-2-ol and apply 25 µl of extract A and 3 portions of 25 µl of extract B at the origin of the plate, as shown in Fig. 5.
3. Apply 10 µl of the respective standard mixtures to the plate, as shown in Fig. 5.

Fig. 5. Thin-layer chromatography drug screening procedure: preparing and spotting the plate

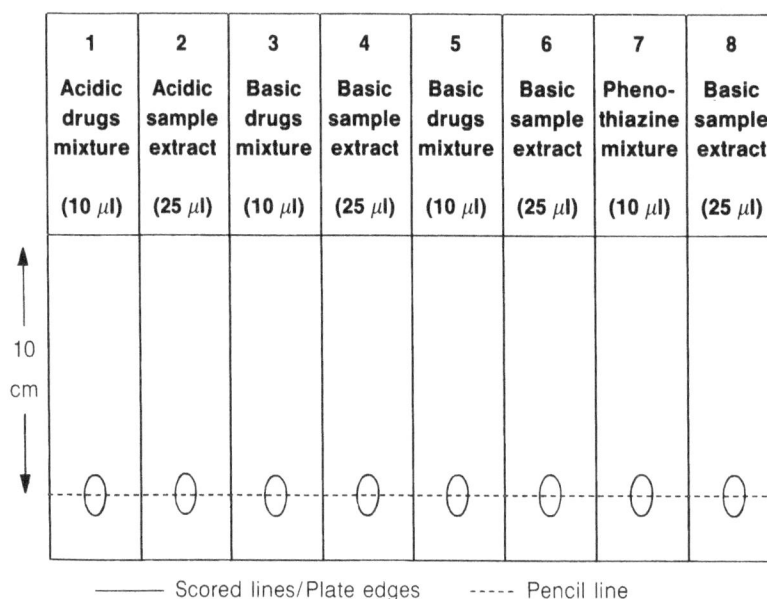

—— Scored lines/Plate edges   ----- Pencil line

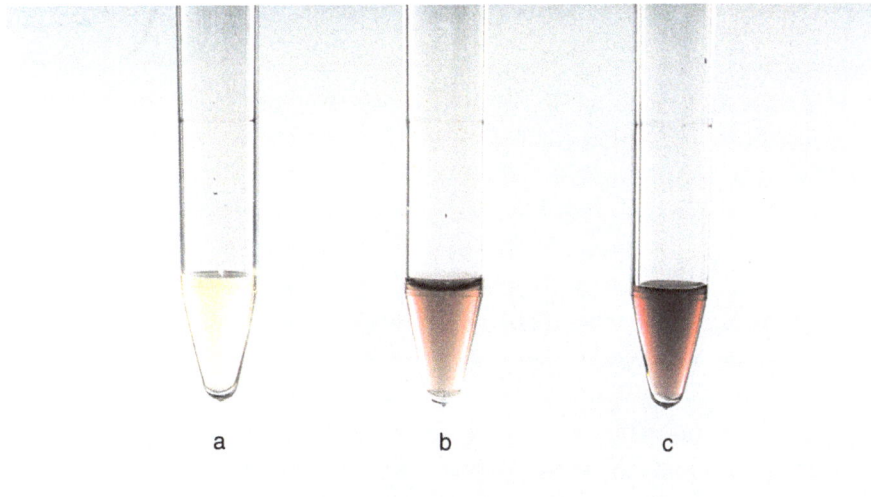

Plate 1. *Qualitative test for salicylic acid (Trinder's test): (a) urine blank, (b) weak positive result, (c) strong positive result.*

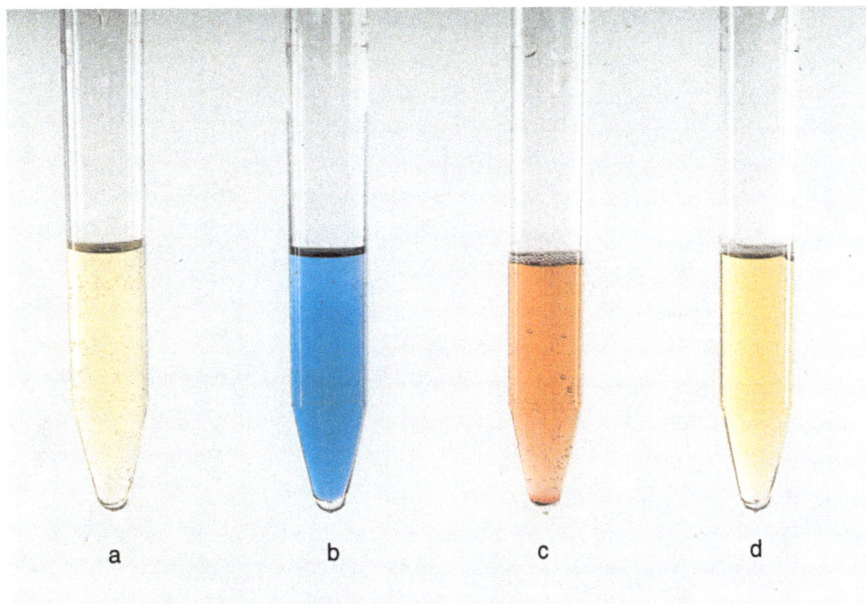

Plate 2. *Qualitative test for phenothiazines (FPN test): (a) blank urine, (b) thioridazine, (c) perphenazine, (d) trifluperazine.*

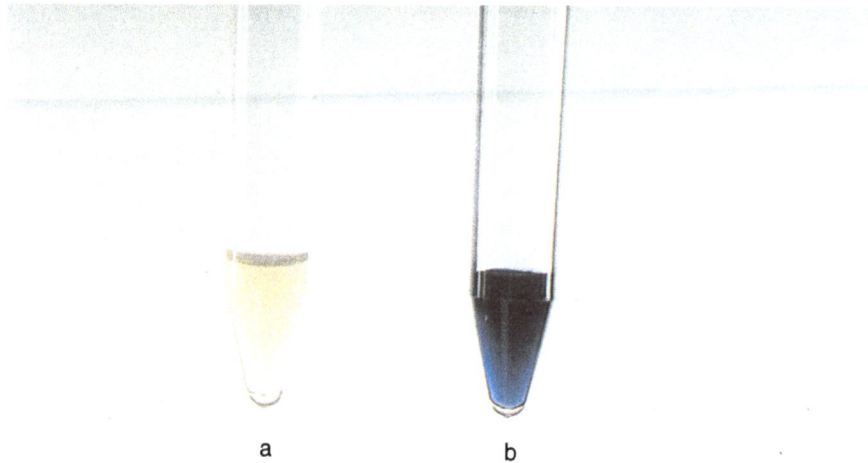

Plate 3. *Qualitative test for imipramine (Forrest test): (a) blank, (b) positive result.*

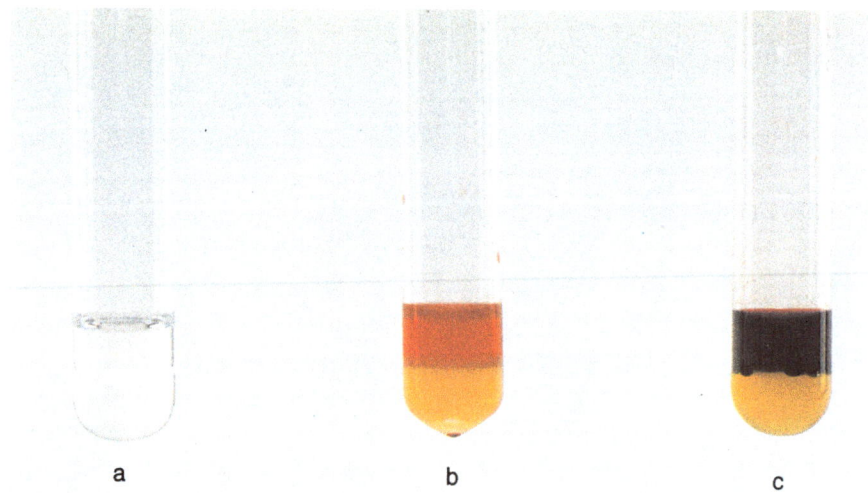

Plate 4. *'Spot' test for trichloro compounds (Fujiwara test) in urine: (a) reagent blank, (b) positive result, and (c) strong positive result.*

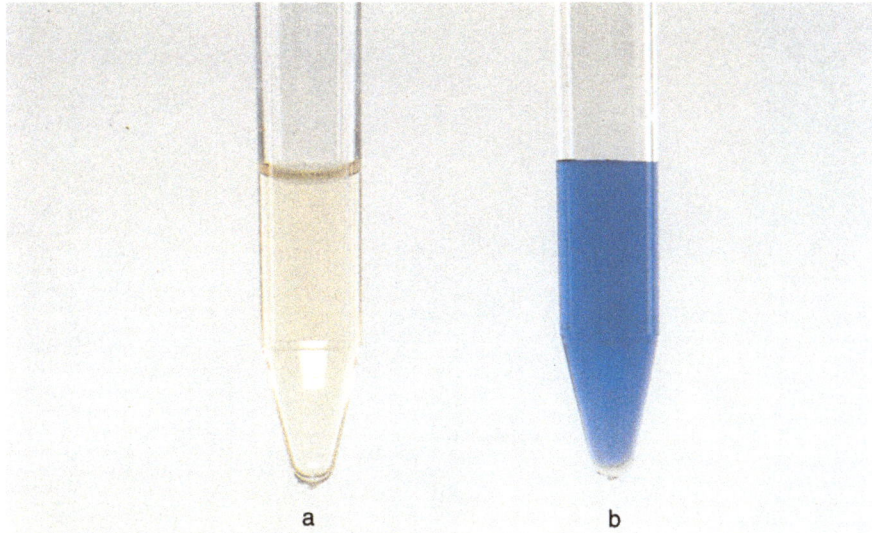

Plate 5. *Qualitative test for paracetamol and phenacetin (o-cresol/ammonia test): (a) blank, and (b) positive result.*

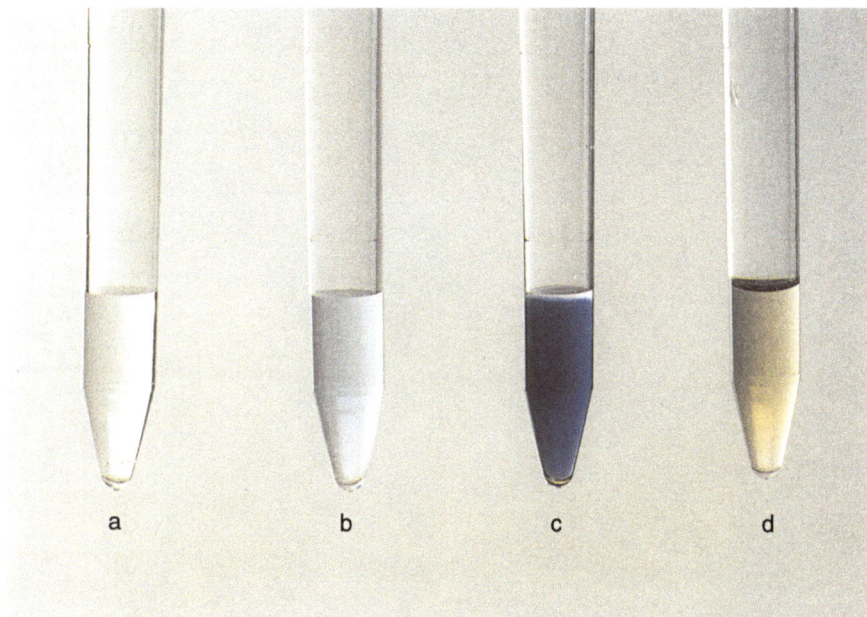

Plate 6. *Qualitative test for paraquat and diquat (dithionite test): (a) reagent blank, (b) weak positive for paraquat, (c) strong positive for paraquat, and (d) weak positive for paraquat in urine sample.*

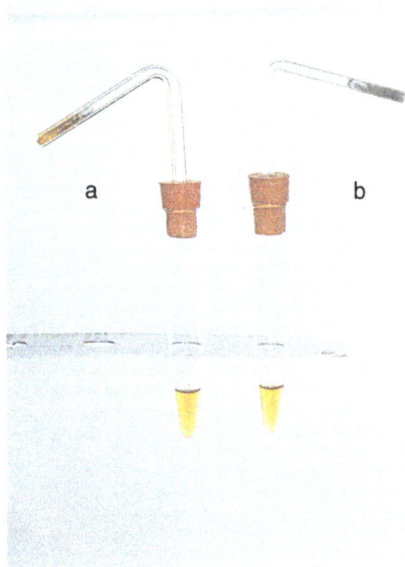

Plate 7. *Qualitative test for volatile reducing substances: (a) blank, (b) positive for ethanol.*

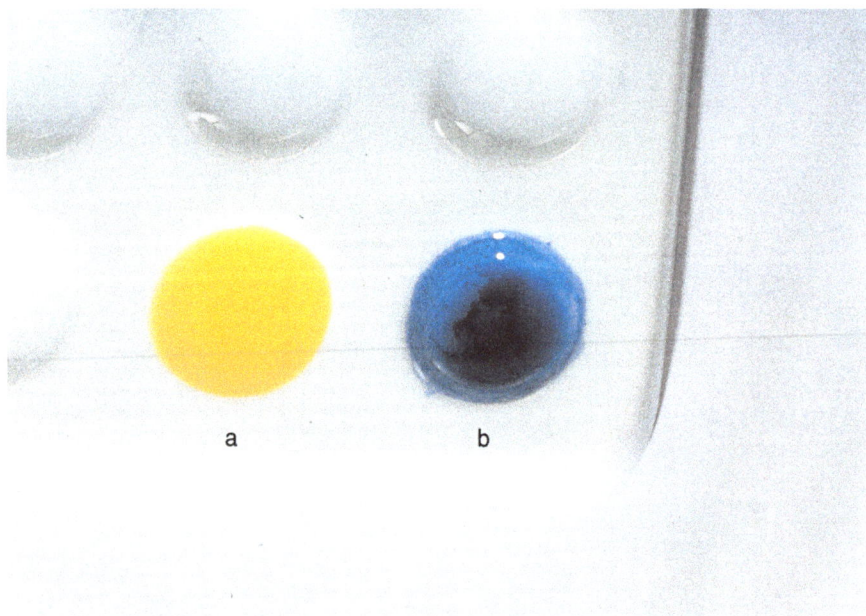

Plate 8. *Qualitative test for ferrous and ferric iron: (a) blank, and (b) positive result. The test has been carried out on a porcelain "spotting" tile.*

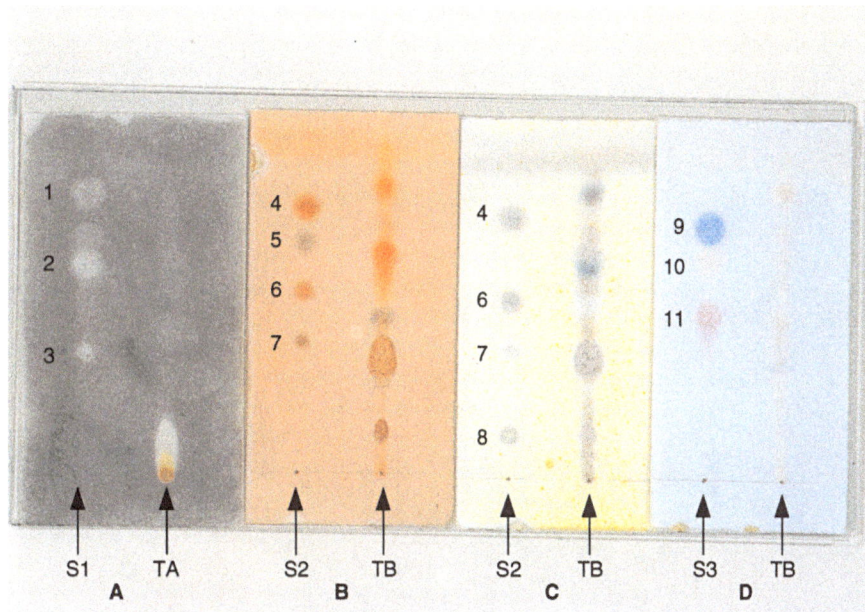

Plate 9. *An example of a chromatogram obtained from the analysis of an acidic and a basic urine extract from a patient following the ingestion of codeine and methadone. The plate is divided into four sections for the application of separate visualization reagents: A–mercurous nitrate; B–acidified iodoplatinate; C–Mandelin's reagent; D–sulfuric acid. The acidic sample extract (TA) has been applied at the origin in section A and run with test mixture S1 containing: amobarbital (1), phenobarbital (2), and theophylline (3). The "basic" extract (TB) has been applied at the origin in sections B, C and D and run with test mixtures: S2 containing amitriptyline (4), nicotine (5), nortriptyline (6), codeine (7), and mefenamic acid (8); and S3 containing thioridazine (9), trifluoperazine (10), and perphenazine (11).*

Note that a complex pattern of drug and metabolites is obtained for the basic sample extract (TB) visualized with iodoplatinate (B) and Mandelin's reagent (C). No response is seen using sulfuric acid (D). No response is seen for the acidic sample extract (TA) visualized using mercurous nitrate in section A.

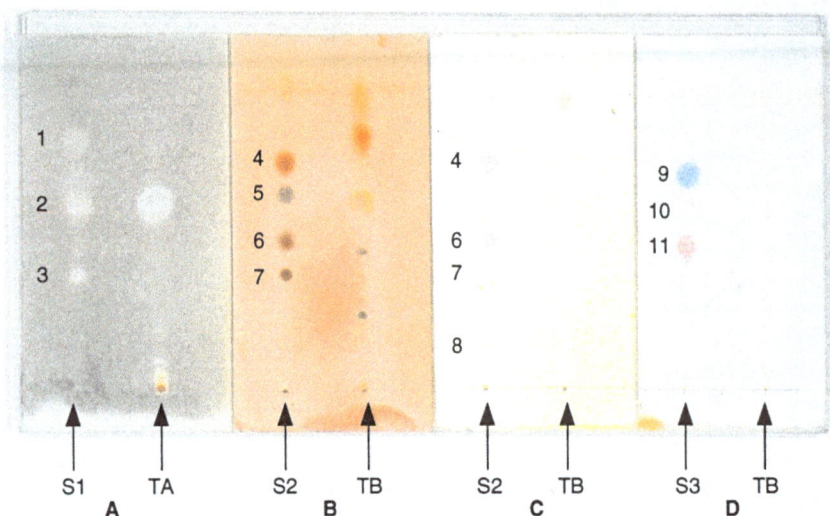

Plate 10. *An example of a chromatogram obtained from the analysis of an acidic and a basic urine extract from a patient following the ingestion of phenobarbital and methadone. The plate is divided into four sections for the application of separate visualization reagents: A — mercurous nitrate; B — acidified iodoplatinate; C — Mandelin's reagent; D – sulfuric acid. The acidic sample extract (TA) has been applied at the origin in section A and run with test mixture S1 containing: amobarbital (1), phenobarbital (2), and theophylline (3). The basic extract (TB) has been applied at the origin in sections B, C and D and run with test mixtures: S2 containing amitriptyline (4), nicotine (5), nortriptyline (6), codeine (7), and mefenamic acid (8); and S3 containing thioridazine (9), trifluoperazine (10), and perphenazine (11).*

Note that the phenobarbital is clearly visualized in the acidic urine extract (TA) using the mercurous nitrate spray (A), whereas methadone and its metabolites are best visualized in the basic urine extract (TB) with iodoplatinate (B). No distinct response is seen with the remaining two sprays, Mandelin's reagent (C) and sulfuric acid (D).

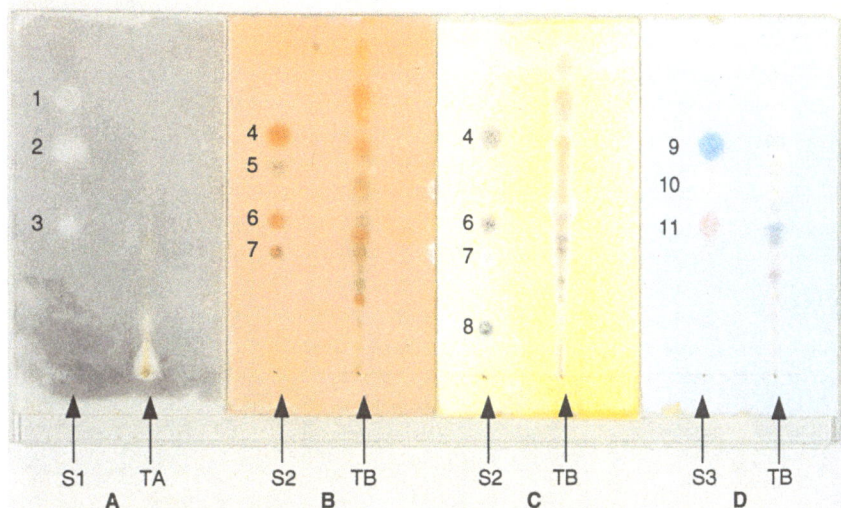

Plate 11. *An example of a chromatogram obtained from the analysis of an acidic and a basic urine extract from a patient following the ingestion of a phenothiazine (thioridazine) overdose. The plate is divided into four sections for the application of separate visualization reagents: A — mercurous nitrate; B — acidified iodoplatinate; C — Mandelin's reagent; D — sulfuric acid. The acidic sample extract (TA) has been applied at the origin in section A and run with test mixture S1 containing: amobarbital (1), phenobarbital (2), and theophylline (3). The basic extract (TB) has been applied at the origin in sections B, C and D and run with test mixtures: S2 containing amitriptyline (4), nicotine (5), nortriptyline (6), codeine (7), and mefenamic acid (8); and S3 containing thioridazine (9), trifluoperazine (10), and perphenazine (11).*

Note that a complex pattern of drug and metabolites is obtained for the basic sample extract (TB) visualized with iodoplatinate (B), Mandelin's reagent (C) and sulfuric acid (D). No response is seen with mercurous nitrate (A) for the acidic sample extract (TA). The pattern of many spots and distinct colours with sulfuric acid is typical of phenothiazine-type compounds, but the pattern is quite dissimilar to that seen for the pure compound (thioridazine).

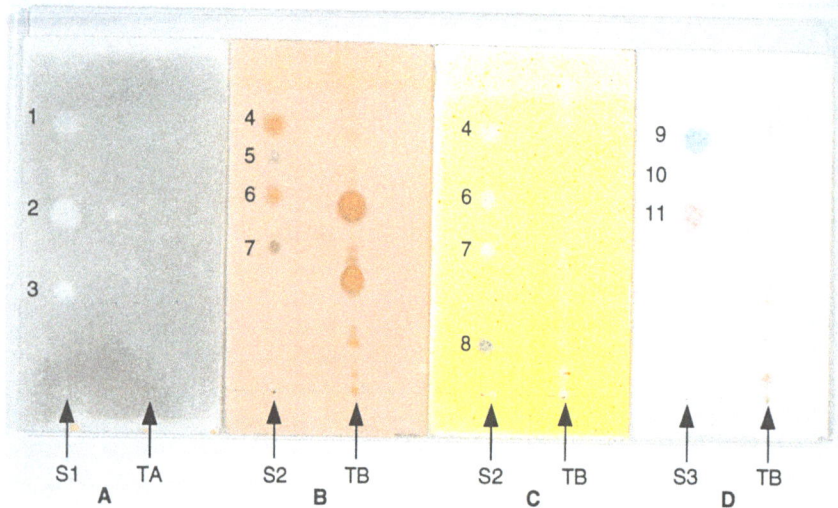

Plate 12. *An example of a chromatogram obtained from the analysis of an acidic and a basic urine extract from a patient following the ingestion of the tricyclic antidepressant, dosulepin. The plate is divided into four sections for the application of separate visualization reagents: A–mercurous nitrate; B–acidified iodoplatinate; C–Mandelin's reagent; D–sulfuric acid. The acidic sample extract (TA) has been applied at the origin in section A and run with test mixture S1 containing: amobarbital (1), phenobarbital (2), and theophylline (3). The basic extract (TB) has been applied at the origin in sections B, C and D and run with test mixtures: S2 containing amitriptyline (4), nicotine (5), nortriptyline (6), codeine (7), and mefenamic acid (8); and S3 containing thioridazine (9), trifluoperazine (10), and perphenazine (11).*

Note that dosulepin and its metabolites are visualized in the basic urine extract (TB) most clearly using the iodoplatinate spray (B). No response is seen with the other sprays (C and D), or with mercurous nitrate spray (A).

Fig. 6. Thin-layer chromatography drug screening procedure: spraying the plate

1	2	3	4	5	6	7	8
Acidic drugs mixture	Acidic sample extract	Basic drugs mixture	Basic sample extract	Basic drugs mixture	Basic sample extract	Pheno-thiazine mixture	Basic sample extract
Mercurous nitrate reagent		Acidified iodoplatinate reagent		Mandelin's reagent		Sulfuric acid (500 ml/l)	

4. Ensure that the plate is dry, and then develop the chromatogram using ethyl acetate:methanol:concentrated ammonium hydroxide (EMA) (saturated tank, see section 4.4.3).
5. Remove the plate and dry under a stream of air **in a fume cupboard or under a fume hood**.
6. View the plate under ultraviolet light (254 nm and 366 nm) and note any fluorescent spots.
7. **Invert the plate** and spray each portion with the visualization reagents as shown in Fig. 6. Take care to mask with a clean glass plate those portions of the plate not being sprayed.

Take care — all the spray reagents used are very toxic. Spraying must be performed in a fume cupboard or under an efficient fume hood.

8. View the plate again under ultraviolet light (254 nm and 366 nm) and note any fluorescent spots, especially in the portion sprayed with Mandelin's reagent.
9. If necessary, the colours obtained with Mandelin's reagent can be enhanced by heating the plate in an oven at 100 °C for 10 minutes.

Results

hR$_f$ values and reactions with the spray reagents of some of the compounds of interest are given in Table 15 and illustrated in Plates 9–12.

Benzodiazepines and their metabolites may appear as light green or yellow spots under ultraviolet light (366 nm) before the mercurous nitrate column (acidic extract) is sprayed, but these compounds are not considered further here (see section 6.11). Quinine (often from bitter drinks), carbamazepine and their metabolites give fluorescent spots (254 nm and 366 nm) before the columns containing the basic extracts are sprayed, and also undergo characteristic reactions with some of the spray reagents. These compounds are relatively easy to identify, as are tricyclic antidepressants (amitriptyline, and imipramine). Others such as nicotine and its metabolites (normally from tobacco), caffeine (from caffeinated beverages) and lidocaine (from catheter lubricant) occur frequently and should be recognizable with practice.

In difficult cases it may be useful to calculate the hR_f value for unknown compounds (section 4.4.5) and to compare the findings with reference values (see Bibliography, p. 234).

Plates 9–12 give some examples of the spot shapes and colours that should be expected for the standards and for some other commonly occurring compounds. Even if the interpretation of the chromatography plate is relatively straightforward, it is important to record systematically the data generated. This can be done by photographing or photocopying the plate (taking great care to clean the photocopier and any other surfaces very carefully afterwards), but it is as easy to record spot positions and shapes on a standard form such as that illustrated in Fig. 7.

Note the position of the yellow-brown streak near the top of the plate observed with Mandelin's reagent (visible light) on analysis of blank urine. Colours, including those observed under ultraviolet light, and any temporal changes, can be noted either in writing or by using coloured pencils.

To ensure reproducible chromatography, attention should be given to the factors discussed in section 4.4.3, especially the use of saturated tanks and the need to ensure that the concentrated ammonium hydroxide is of adequate strength (relative density 0.88, 330 g/l), both in the tank and in the reagent bottle. It is good practice to buy either small (500-ml) bottles or to transfer the contents of large (2.5-litre) bottles of ammonium hydroxide to 500-ml bottles (**with care**), which can be kept tightly stoppered until needed. **Never** use a batch of ethyl acetate:methanol:concentrated ammonium hydroxide mobile phase more than five times at room temperatures of 20–25 °C (fewer times at higher ambient temperatures).

Even when all due precautions are taken, it is invariably found that the chromatographic characteristics of sample extracts are different from those of pure compounds. In extreme cases, broad streaks may be obtained rather than discrete spots. This is often attributable to the presence of polyethylene glycol used as a vehicle in, for example,

Fig. 7. Thin-layer chromatography drug screening procedure: recording the data

Plate: *20 × 20 cm silica gel*   Eluent: *EMA, saturated tank*

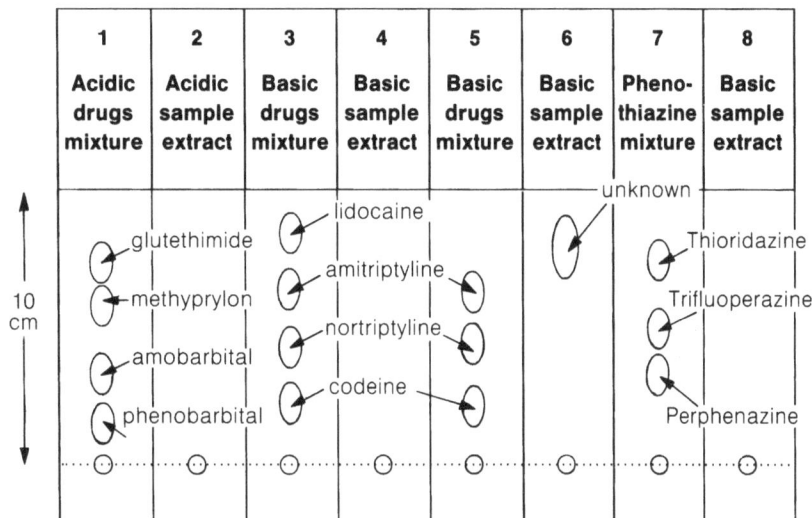

1	2	3	4	5	6	7	8
Acidic drugs mixture	Acidic sample extract	Basic drugs mixture	Basic sample extract	Basic drugs mixture	Basic sample extract	Pheno-thiazine mixture	Basic sample extract

Patient: Analyst:

Sample: Date of analysis:

Date: Time of analysis:

Time: Comments: *To illustrate separation of standards and position of unknown spot often seen with Mandelin's reagent.*
Laboratory no: (Note: the standards illustrated here are not necessarily those shown in the colour plates.)

temazepam capsules and can be minimized by back-extraction of acidic or basic compounds into dilute base or acid, respectively, as described above.

Sensitivity

It is not possible to give detection limits for all the compounds under study. The experience of the analyst, the extraction efficiency, the spot density, the intensity of the chromogenic reaction with the spray reagents and even the type of silica gel used can all affect sensitivity. Nevertheless, a general limit of sensitivity of 1 mg/l is reasonable.

5.2.4 *Reporting the results*

The results of emergency analyses must be communicated direct to the clinician without delay, and should be followed by a written report as

Fig. 8. Example of an analytical toxicology report form

ANALYTICAL TOXICOLOGY REPORT	General comments/Clinical interpretation:
From: [Insert laboratory name, address and telephone no.] Signed: Date:	
Patient: First name: Age/Date of birth: Sex: Consultant: Ward: Reference no:	

Sample type	Date	Time	Laboratory no	Analytical findings	Concentration	Method used

soon as possible. An example of an analytical toxicology report form is given in Fig. 8. Ideally, confirmation using a second, independent method, or failing this an independent duplicate, should be obtained before positive findings are reported. However, this may not always be practicable, especially if only simple methods are available. In such cases it is vital that the appropriate positive and negative controls have been analysed together with the specimen (see section 4.1.5).

When reporting quantitative results it is important to state clearly the units of measurement used (SI mass units are preferable; see section 4.1.6). In addition, any information necessary to ensure that the clinical implications of the result are fully understood should be noted on the written report. The clinical features associated with poisoning by a number of compounds are given in the appropriate monographs (section 6). Information on additional compounds will usually be found in one of the clinical toxicology textbooks listed in the Bibliography (p. 234).

Although it is often easy for the analyst to interpret the results of analyses in which no compounds are detected, such results are sometimes difficult to convey to clinicians, especially in writing. It is important to give information as to the poisons **excluded** by the tests performed with all the attendant complications of the scope, sensitivity and selectivity of the analyses, and other factors such as sampling variations. Because of the potential medicolegal and other implications of any toxicological analysis, it is important **not** to use laboratory jargon such as "negative" or sweeping statements such as "absent" or "not present".

The phrase "not detected" should convey precisely the laboratory result, especially when accompanied by a description of the specimen analysed and the limit of sensitivity of the test (detection limit). However, it can still be difficult to convey the scope of analyses, such as the thin-layer chromatography screen for acidic and basic drugs discussed above. Even with Trinder's test for example, — a relatively simple test normally used to detect acetylsalicylic acid ingestion (Table 14) — a number of other salicylates including, of course, salicylic acid itself also react. One way of giving at least some of this information in a written report is to list the compounds or groups of compounds normally detected by commonly used procedures. If these groups are

Table 16. Qualitative test groups (see also Fig. 3)

Group	Compounds
1	Salicylates (including acetylsalicylic acid (aspirin), 4-aminosalicylic acid, methyl salicylate and salicylic acid)
2	Phenothiazines (including chlorpromazine, perphenazine, prochlorperazine, promazine, promethazine and thioridazine)
3	Imipramine and related compounds (including clomipramine, desipramine and trimipramine)
4	Trichloro compounds (including chloral hydrate, chloroform, dichloralphenazone and trichloroethylene
5	Paracetamol
6	Paraquat and diquat
7	Volatile reducing agents (including ethanol and methanol)
8	Strong oxidizing agents (including bromates, chlorates, hypochlorites, nitrates and nitrites)
9	Iron
10a	TLC acidic drugs (including barbiturates, glutethimide, methyprylon, phenytoin and primidone)
10b	TLC basic drugs (including antihistamines (cyclizine and diphenhydramine), antimalarials (chloroquine and quinine), amfetamine, atropine, caffeine, carbamazepine, cardioactive drugs (lidocaine, propranolol, quinidine, and verapamil), clomethiazole, cocaine, ephedrine, haloperidol, methaqualone, opioids (codeine, dextropropoxyphene, diamorphine, dihydrocodeine, methadone, morphine and pethidine), orphenadrine, phenothiazines (chlorpromazine, perphenazine, prochlorperazine, promazine, promethazine and thioridazine), strychnine and tricyclic antidepressants (amitriptyline, clomipramine, doxepin, desipramine, dosulepin, imipramine, nortriptyline, protriptyline and trimipramine))

listed on the back of the report then it is relatively simple to refer to the qualitative tests performed by number and thus to convey at least some of the information required. An example of a grouping system based on that used in the analytical toxicology laboratory worksheet (see Fig. 3) is given in Table 16.

5.2.5 *Summary*

It should be clear that performing a qualitative poisons screen involves more than simply analysing specimens as they arrive in the laboratory and reporting the bare facts of the analysis. The suggested scheme of operation is summarized in Table 17.

Table 17. Summary of the suggested analytical scheme

Step	Action
1	Assess urgency and nature of request. Confirm and record clinical details (see Fig. 2). Advise on collection of specimens.
2	Check details of the specimens received, particularly dates and times in relation to suspected date and time of ingestion.
3	Carry out preliminary physical examination of samples and scene residues (section 5.2.1)
4	Perform simple tests for specific compounds if indicated by history or clinical examination (section 6). Also, if indicated by the history, perform quantitative measurements using plasma, serum or whole blood. Record results using laboratory worksheet (see Fig. 3).
5	Carry out direct qualitative tests on urine, stomach contents or scene residues (sections 5.2.2 and 5.2.3). Record the results using laboratory worksheet (see Fig. 3).
6	Prepare acidic and basic extracts of the sample for TLC (section 5.2.3). Spot sample extracts and standards (sample extracts first) and develop TLC plates in ethyl acetate: methanol: concentrated ammonium hydroxide (85:10:5) (EMA).
7	Dry the plate and visualize the chromatogram in the sequence: (*a*) ultraviolet (254 nm and 366 nm), (*b*) spray reagents, and (*c*) ultraviolet (254 nm and 366 nm).
8	Collate the results and prepare a written record as soon as possible (see Fig. 7). Are the results in keeping with the clinical condition of the patient (feasibility control)?
9	Perform quantitative measurements using plasma/serum or whole blood if indicated. Carry out any necessary additional tests on the original, or additional, samples.
10	Telephone urgent results to clinical staff, taking care to ensure that they are written down and that the clinical implications are fully understood. Issue written report (see Fig. 8).

Monographs — analytical and toxicological data

These monographs give practical information on detecting and identifying some common poisons or groups of poisons (see Table 1). In order to simplify presentation, no original references have been given, but further details on individual entries are available in the references listed in the Bibliography (p. 234). Reference is made as appropriate to specific aspects of laboratory practice (section 4) and to the poisons screening procedure (section 5.2). As noted previously, this procedure should usually be followed when there is no clinical or circumstantial evidence as to the poison(s) involved in a particular case.

6.1 Amfetamine

α-Methylphenethylamine; $C_9H_{13}N$; relative molecular mass, 135

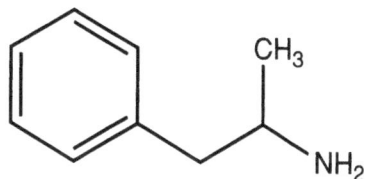

Amfetamine and its *N*-methyl analogue, metamfetamine, are central nervous system stimulants and are widely abused.

There is no simple qualitative test for amfetamine, but this and other similar compounds can be detected and identified by thin-layer chromatography of a basic solvent extract of urine, stomach contents or scene residues. However, the extract **must** be acidified by addition of 0.5 ml of methanolic hydrochloric acid (2 ml/l) to prevent loss of volatile bases at the evaporation stage, as noted in section 5.2.3.

Clinical interpretation

Oral or intravenous amfetamine overdosage may cause hyperthermia, convulsions, coma, and respiratory and/or cardiac failure, but death from acute amfetamine poisoning is comparatively rare. Treatment is generally symptomatic and supportive. Quantitative measurements in blood are not normally required in management.

6.2 Aminophenazone

Amidopyrine, aminopyrine, 4-dimethylamino-1,5-dimethyl-2-phenyl-4-pyrazolin-3-one; $C_{13}H_{17}N_3O$; relative molecular mass, 231.

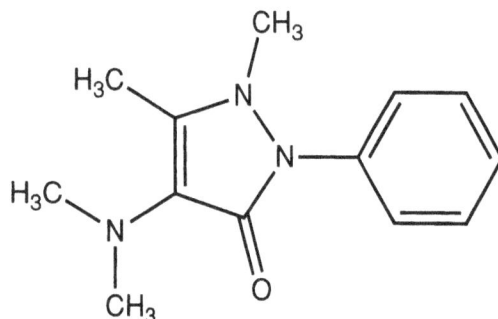

Aminophenazone is an analgesic and antipyretic which is now little used since agranulocytosis and renal tubular necrosis may occur after therapeutic dosage. Ingestion of about 10 g can cause severe acute poisoning in an adult.

Qualitative test

Applicable to urine, stomach contents and scene residues.

Reagents
1. Aqueous sodium hydroxide (1 mol/l).
2. Aqueous silver nitrate solution (100 g/l).
3. Aqueous hydrochloric acid (5 mol/l).
4. Potassium nitrite (solid).

Method
1. Add 1 ml of sodium hydroxide solution to 5 ml of sample and add 10 ml of chloroform.
2. Extract on a mechanical shaker for 5 minutes, centrifuge and discard the upper aqueous phase.
3. Filter the chloroform extract through phase-separating filter-paper (see section 4.3.2) into a clean tube, evaporate to dryness under a stream of compressed air or nitrogen, and reconstitute the residue in 1 ml of purified water.
4. Add 0.5 ml of silver nitrate solution to 0.5 ml of the reconstituted extract.
5. Add 1 ml of hydrochloric acid and about 1 mg of solid potassium nitrite to the remaining portion of the extract.

Results

On addition of silver nitrate (step 4), a blue solution which turns black on standing indicates aminophenazone. In step 5, potassium nitrite imparts a blue-violet colour which quickly fades.

Aminophenazone can also be detected by thin-layer chromatography of a basic extract of urine, stomach contents or scene residues (section 5.2.3), and this should always be performed in addition to the test given above.

Sensitivity

Aminophenazone, 50 mg/l.

Clinical interpretation

Aminophenazone overdosage may cause hypotension, convulsions, and delirium. Treatment is symptomatic and supportive. Quantitative measurements in blood are not required in management.

6.3 Amitriptyline

3-(10,11-Dihydro-5*H*-dibenzo[*a,d*]cyclohepten-5-ylidene)-*N*,*N*-dimethylpropylamine; $C_{20}H_{23}N$; relative molecular mass, 277

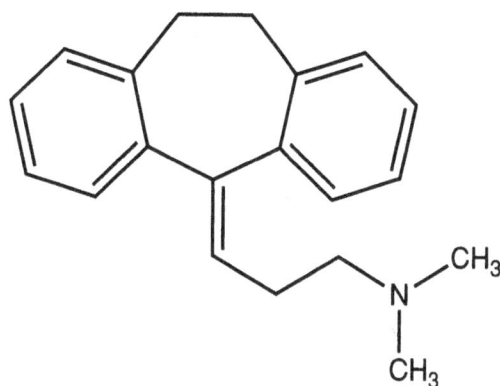

Amitriptyline is a widely used tricyclic antidepressant. It is metabolized by *N*-demethylation to nortriptyline, which is an antidepressant in its own right. Protriptyline is an analogue of amitriptyline.

There is no simple qualitative test for amitriptyline, but this compound and other tricyclic antidepressants can be easily detected and identified by thin-layer chromatography of a basic solvent extract of urine, stomach contents or scene residues (see section 5.2.3).

Clinical interpretation

Acute poisoning with amitriptyline and other tricyclic antidepressants may cause dilated pupils, hypotension, hypothermia, cardiac arrhythmias, depressed respiration, coma, convulsions and cardiorespiratory arrest. Urinary retention is also a feature of poisoning with these compounds, and this may delay procurement of an appropriate specimen for analysis.

Treatment is generally symptomatic and supportive. The use of antiarrhythmic agents should generally be avoided, but alkalinization using sodium bicarbonate may be employed. Quantitative measurements in blood are not normally required in management.

6.4 Aniline

Phenylamine; $C_6H_5NH_2$; relative molecular mass, 93

Aniline is used mainly as an intermediate in the manufacture of dyes and other chemicals. It is metabolized to p-aminophenol and p-acetamidophenol, which are excreted in urine as sulfate and glucuronide conjugates. On hydrolysis of urine, p-aminophenol is reformed, and can be detected using the o-cresol/ammonia test. Aniline and other primary aromatic amines form diazo compounds with nitrous acid, which couple with 1-naphthylethylenediamine to form highly coloured derivatives. This reaction forms the basis of the confirmatory test described below.

Qualitative test

Applicable to urine. o-Cresol/ammonia test.

Reagents

1. Concentrated hydrochloric acid (relative density 1.18).
2. Aqueous o-cresol (10 g/l).
3. Aqueous ammonium hydroxide (4 mol/l).

Method

1. Add 0.5 ml of hydrochloric acid to 0.5 ml of sample, boil for 10 minutes and cool.
2. Add 1 ml of o-cresol solution to 0.2 ml of the hydrolysate.
3. Add 2 ml of ammonium hydroxide solution and mix for 5 seconds.

Results

A strong, royal blue colour developing rapidly indicates the presence of p-aminophenol. Metabolites of paracetamol (and thus phenacetin) and nitrobenzene also give *p*-aminophenol on hydrolysis and so interfere. Ethylenediamine (from aminophylline, for example; see section 6.105) gives a green colour in this test.

Sensitivity

p-Aminophenol, 10 mg/l.

Confirmatory test

Applicable to stomach contents and scene residues.

Reagents

1. Aqueous sodium nitrite solution (2 g/l, freshly prepared).
2. Aqueous hydrochloric acid (2 mol/l).
3. Aqueous ammonium sulfamate solution (10 g/l).
4. Aqueous *N*-(1-naphthyl)ethylenediamine dihydrochloride solution (2 g/l, freshly prepared).

Method

1. Mix 0.1 ml of sodium nitrite solution and 0.2 ml of dilute hydrochloric acid in a 5-ml test-tube.
2. Add 0.1 ml of sample, mix and allow to stand for 2 minutes.
3. Add 0.2 ml of ammonium sulfamate solution followed by 0.1 ml of *N*-(1-naphthyl)ethylenediamine dihydrochloride solution.

Results

A purple colour after 1 minute indicates the presence of aniline.

Sensitivity

Aniline, 10 mg/l.

Clinical interpretation

Poisoning with aniline usually results from inhalation or dermal absorption. Symptoms occur within 1–3 hours of exposure and include confusion, nausea, vomiting and diarrhoea, with convulsions, coma and hepatic and renal damage in severe cases. Haemolysis, red (wine)-coloured urine, and methaemoglobinaemia (dark chocolate-coloured blood) may also occur (section 3.2.2). Blood methaemoglobin can be measured but is unstable and the use of stored samples is unreliable. Hepatic and renal function tests are essential, however. Treatment may include intravenous methylene blue, but this is contraindicated in patients with glucose-6-phosphate dehydrogenase deficiency, since there is a high risk of inducing haemolysis.

6.5 Antimony

Trivalent and pentavalent salts of antimony (Sb) are used parenterally in the treatment of schistosomiasis and leishmaniasis. Antimony salts are also used in pigments and abrasives and for flame-proofing fabrics. As with arsenic, bismuth and mercury, antimony can be detected using the Reinsch test.

Qualitative test

Applicable to urine, stomach contents and scene residues.

Reagents

1. Concentrated hydrochloric acid (relative density 1.18).
2. Aqueous hydrochloric acid (2 mol/l).
3. Copper foil or mesh (5 × 10 mm) or wire (2–3 cm).
4. Aqueous nitric acid (500 ml/l).

Method

1. Immediately before use, clean the foil, mesh or wire in nitric acid until the copper acquires a bright surface.
2. Rinse the copper with purified water and add 10 ml of concentrated hydrochloric acid and 20 ml of test solution in a 100-ml conical flask.
3. Heat on a boiling water-bath **in a fume cupboard** for 1 hour. Maintain the volume of the solution by adding dilute hydrochloric acid as necessary.
4. Cool and gently wash the copper with purified water.

Results

Staining on the copper can be interpreted as follows:

purple black — antimony
dull black — arsenic
shiny black — bismuth
silvery — mercury

Selenium and tellurium may also give dark deposits, while high concentrations of sulfur may give a speckled appearance to the copper.

An estimation of the concentration of antimony in the sample can be made by comparison of the deposit on the copper with that obtained from a solution containing a known concentration of the element.

Sensitivity

Antimony, about 2 mg/l.

Confirmatory test

Applicable to the stained (purple black) copper from the test above.

Reagents

1. Aqueous potassium cyanide solution (100 g/l). **Take care when using concentrated cyanide solutions**.
2. Aqueous sodium sulfite solution (50 g/l, freshly prepared).
3. Aqueous nitric acid (3 mol/l).
4. Quinine/potassium iodide reagent. Dissolve 1 g of quinine sulfate in 100 ml of purified water containing 0.5 ml of concentrated nitric acid (relative density 1.42). When the quinine has completely dissolved, add 2 g of potassium iodide.

Method

1. Place the copper in potassium cyanide solution and leave for 10 minutes.
2. Wash any undissolved stain with purified water and add 1 ml of sodium sulfite solution and 1 ml of aqueous nitric acid.
3. Agitate frequently for 5 minutes and add 1 ml of purified water and 1 ml of quinine/potassium iodide reagent.

Results

Stains due to arsenic dissolve in potassium cyanide solution, while stains due to bismuth and antimony do not. Bismuth slowly forms an orange/brown suspension with quinine/potassium iodide.

Sensitivity

Antimony, about 2 mg/l.

Clinical interpretation

Parenteral administration of antimony salts may lead to cardiotoxicity; collapse and death from anaphylactic shock may also occur. Industrial poisoning is usually due to inhalation of antimony compounds either as fumes or dusts. The symptoms of acute oral antimony poisoning resemble those of acute arsenic poisoning and include abdominal pain, vomiting and diarrhoea. The measurement of blood antimony concentrations is useful in diagnosing acute poisoning, but this requires atomic absorption spectrophotometry.

6.6 Arsenic

A number of pesticides contain arsenic (As) in the form of arsenic acid, dimethylarsenic acid, and arsenite, arsenate and methanearsonate salts.

Arsenical compounds are also used in pharmaceuticals and in the manufacture of ceramics and glass. Arsine (AsH_3) gas is used in certain industrial processes and may also be liberated accidentally from other arsenical products.

As with antimony, bismuth and mercury, arsenic can be detected and identified using the Reinsch test. The method described below for the quantitative assay to measure urinary arsenic concentrations is a modified Gutzeit procedure. In summary, arsine is generated by reaction of arsenic-containing compounds in the sample with nascent hydrogen. The arsine is carried in a stream of hydrogen through a lead acetate-impregnated filter (to remove sulfides), and arsenic is trapped in a bubbler by a solution of silver diethyldithiocarbamate in pyridine.

Qualitative test

Applicable to urine, stomach contents and scene residues.
Reinsch test — see antimony monograph (section 6.5).

Results

Staining on the copper can be interpreted as follows:

purple black — antimony
dull black — arsenic
shiny black — bismuth
silvery — mercury

Selenium and tellurium may also give dark deposits, while high concentrations of sulfur may give a speckled appearance to the copper.

An estimation of the concentration of arsenic in the sample can be made by comparison of the deposit on the copper with that obtained from a solution containing a known concentration of the element.

Sensitivity

Arsenic, about 5 mg/l.

Confirmatory test

Applicable to the stained (dull black) copper from the test above.

Reagent

Aqueous potassium cyanide solution (100 g/l). **Take care when using concentrated cyanide solutions**.

Method

Place the copper in potassium cyanide solution and leave for 10 minutes.

Results

Arsenical stains dissolve in potassium cyanide solution while stains due to bismuth and antimony do not.

Sensitivity

Arsenic, about 5 mg/l.

Quantitative assay

Applicable to urine.

Reagents

1. Silver diethyldithiocarbamate solution (5 g/l) in pyridine.
2. Aqueous lead acetate solution (200 g/l).
3. Stannous chloride (330 g/l) in aqueous hydrochloric acid (200 ml/l).
4. Concentrated hydrochloric acid (relative density 1.18).
5. Potassium iodide (solid).
6. Granulated zinc.

Apparatus

Modified Gutzeit apparatus (Fig. 9).

Standards

Dissolve 2.4 g of arsenic trichloride in 1 litre of dilute hydrochloric acid (1 mol/l); this gives a solution containing an arsenic concentration of 1 g/l. Dilute with purified water to give solutions containing arsenic concentrations of 0.5, 2.0, 5.0 and 10.0 mg/l.

Method

1. Clean the modified Gutzeit apparatus with acetone and dry.
2. Soak a plug of glass wool in lead acetate solution and allow to dry at room temperature.
3. Insert the treated glass wool into the top (capillary) end of the guard tube.
4. Introduce 3.0 ml of silver diethyldithiocarbamate solution into the bubbler.
5. Add 2 g of potassium iodide and 50 ml of sample to the 100-ml conical flask, swirl until dissolved, and add 2 ml of stannous chloride solution and 10 ml of concentrated hydrochloric acid.
6. Mix well, add 10 g of granulated zinc and quickly position the bubbler and check the seals of all joints.
7. Allow the reaction to proceed for 45 minutes at room temperature.

Fig. 9. Modified Gutzeit apparatus (after Fisher Scientific)

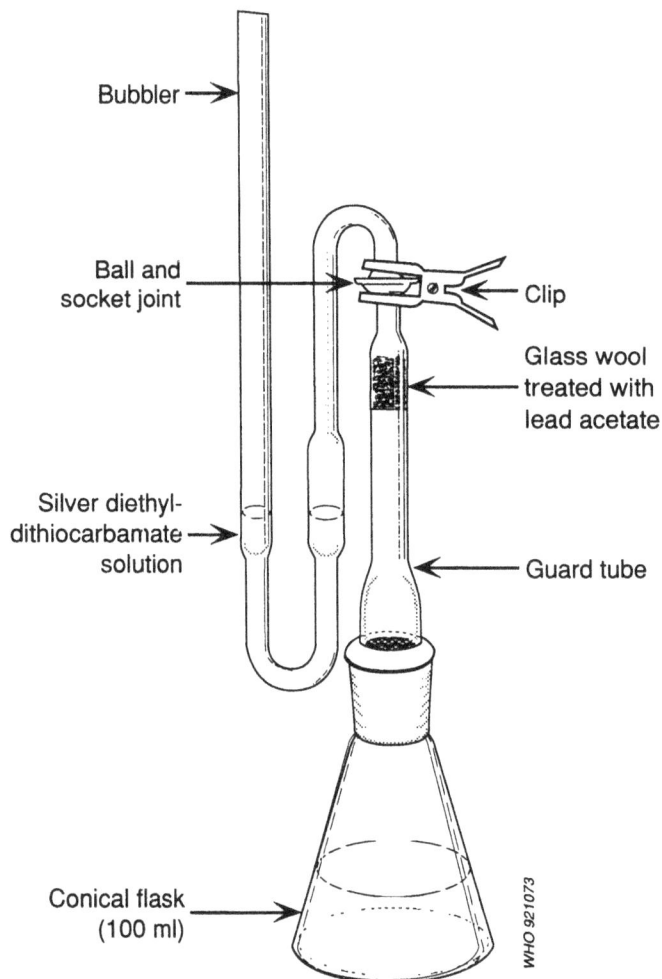

8. Disconnect the bubbler and swirl gently to dissolve any complex formed on the walls and to mix the solution thoroughly.

Results

Measure the absorbance of the solution at 540 nm against a reagent blank (see section 4.5.2) and calculate the arsenic concentration using a previously prepared calibration graph. The calibration is linear for arsenic concentrations up to 10 mg/l. Germanium and antimony interfere in this assay.

Sensitivity

Arsenic, 0.5 mg/l.

Clinical interpretation

Acute ingestion of arsenical salts produces severe abdominal pain, vomiting and copious, bloody diarrhoea. Death from circulatory collapse often ensues. Inhalation of arsine produces massive haemolysis and renal failure. Treatment with chelating agents may be indicated.

6.7 Atenolol

2-[4-(2-Hydroxy-3-isopropylaminopropoxy)phenyl] acetamide; $C_{14}H_{22}N_2O_3$; relative molecular mass, 266

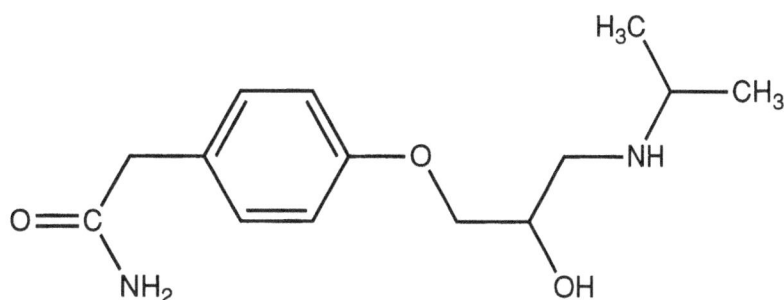

Atenolol is a cardio-selective β-adrenoceptor blocking agent (β-blocker) used in the treatment of hypertension.

There is no simple qualitative test for atenolol, but it can be detected and identified by thin-layer chromatography of a basic solvent extract of urine, stomach contents or scene residues (see section 5.2.3).

Clinical interpretation

In acute overdose, atenolol may cause bronchoconstriction, hypotension and cardiac failure. Treatment is symptomatic and supportive, and may include the use of β-agonists. Quantitative measurements in blood are not normally required in management.

6.8 Atropine

(1R,3r,5S)-Tropan-3-yl(±)-tropate, $C_{17}H_{23}NO_3$; relative molecular mass 289

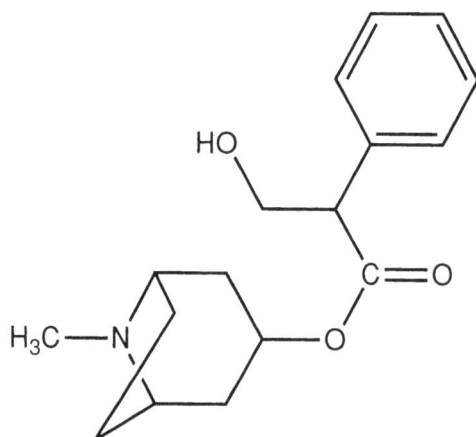

Atropine occurs in plants such as *Atropa belladonna* and *Datura stramonium*. It has potent anticholinergic activity and is used to reduce bronchial and salivary secretions before anaesthesia, to treat gastrointestinal spasm and to produce mydriasis in ophthalmic procedures. Atropine is also used as an antidote to poisoning with inhibitors of cholinesterase, such as some organophosphorus pesticides, carbamate pesticides and some chemical warfare agents. Atropine is very potent and doses of 10 mg or more can cause severe poisoning.

There is no simple qualitative test for atropine, but it can be detected and identified by thin-layer chromatography of a basic solvent extract of stomach contents or scene residues (see section 5.2.3). It may also be possible to detect atropine in urine using this procedure, but urinary concentrations are often very low even after overdosage.

Clinical interpretation

Acute atropine overdose may cause tachycardia, hypertension, pyrexia, delirium and hallucinations. Physostigmine is an effective antidote. Quantitative measurements in blood are of no value in management.

6.9 Barbiturates

Barbiturates are 5,5'-disubstituted derivatives of barbituric acid. In addition, the nitrogen atom at position 1 may be methylated as in methylphenobarbital, while substitution of sulfur for oxygen at position 2 gives thiobarbiturates such as thiopental.

The structure of barbituric acid is shown below:

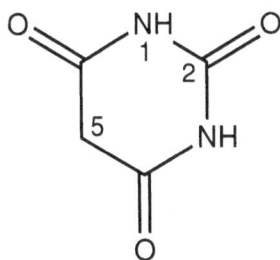

Some commonly occurring barbiturates are listed in Table 18. Other barbiturates that may be encountered include cyclobarbital, cyclopentobarbital, heptabarbital, hexobarbital, methohexital and vinbarbital. Note that barbituric acid itself is no longer used as a drug.

Barbiturates are potent hypnotics and sedatives, but in many countries only phenobarbital and (intravenous) thiopental find wide application nowadays. Barbiturates may also be used for euthanasia in veterinary medicine, and barbital sodium is used as a laboratory chemical, especially in buffer solutions.

In acute poisoning it may be important to ascertain whether barbital or phenobarbital (so-called long-acting barbiturates), or a short- or medium-acting compound has been taken. This is because alkaline diuresis (see section 2.2.3) can enhance the excretion of barbital and phenobarbital, but not of other barbiturates.

Table 18. Some barbiturate hypnotics

Compound	Chemical name	Relative molecular mass
Amobarbital	5-Ethyl-5-isopentylbarbituric acid	226
Barbital	5,5-Diethylbarbituric acid	184
Pentobarbital	5-Ethyl-5(1-methylbutyl)barbituric acid	226
Phenobarbital	5-Ethyl-5-phenylbarbituric acid	232
Secbutabarbital	5-*n*-Butyl-5-ethylbarbituric acid	212
Secobarbital	5-Allyl-5-(1-methylbutyl)barbituric acid	238
Thiopental	5-Ethyl-5-(1-methylbutyl)-2-thiobarbituric acid	242

There is no reliable simple test for these compounds and a qualitative analysis is best performed by thin-layer chromatography of a solvent extract of urine, stomach contents or scene residues (see section 5.2.3). This should also permit identification of the type of barbiturate present, if not the actual compound ingested.

The method given below will permit measurement of total barbiturate in a solvent extract of the specimen, and relies on the characteristic spectral shift shown by barbiturates on going from pH 11 to pH 2. However, ideally a double-beam spectrophotometer is required (see section 4.5). Accurate measurement of individual barbiturates normally requires gas-liquid or high-performance liquid chromatography.

Quantitative assay

Applicable to whole blood, plasma or serum (5 ml).

Reagents

1. Borate buffer, pH 8.4. Mix 22.4 g of disodium tetraborate with 76 ml of aqueous hydrochloric acid (1 mol/l) and dilute to 2 litres with purified water.
2. Aqueous hydrochloric acid (2 mol/l).
3. Concentrated sulfuric acid (relative density 1.83).
4. Concentrated ammonium hydroxide (relative density 0.88).
5. Sodium sulfate/charcoal mixture. Add 100 mg of activated charcoal to 100 g of anhydrous sodium sulfate, mix thoroughly and heat in an evaporating basin at 100 °C for 8 hours. Allow to cool and store in a tightly stoppered bottle.

Standards

Solutions containing barbital at concentrations of 5, 10, 25 and 50 mg/l in blank human plasma, prepared by dilution from an aqueous solution of barbital sodium (1.12 g/l, equivalent to diethylbarbituric acid at a concentration of 1.00 g/l).

Method

1. Add 5 ml of sample, 2 ml of hydrochloric acid and 60 ml of diethyl ether (with care) to a 250-ml separating funnel.
2. Lubricate the stopper of the funnel with purified water, insert and shake gently for 2 minutes.
3. Allow to stand for 5 minutes, and then discard the lower, aqueous phase through the tap of the separating funnel.

4. Add the diethyl ether extract to 10 ml of borate buffer in a second separating funnel and mix for 1 minute.

5. Allow to stand for 5 minutes and again discard the lower, aqueous phase through the funnel tap.

6. Wash round the funnel with 5 ml of purified water, allow to stand for 5 minutes and again discard the lower, aqueous phase through the funnel tap.

7. Add about 4 g of sodium sulfate/charcoal mixture to the ether extract in the funnel, shake to disperse, and filter the extract through phase-separating filter-paper into a 150-ml conical flask.

8. Add a further 20 ml of diethyl ether to the separating funnel, shake and add to the extract in the flask through the filter funnel.

9. Evaporate the extract to dryness on a water-bath at 40 °C under a stream of compressed air or nitrogen.

10. Add 5.0 ml of purified water to the dry extract in the flask, swirl gently and allow to stand for 5 minutes.

11. Filter the reconstituted extract through phase-separating filter-paper into a 12.5-cm test-tube.

12. Check the spectrophotometer zero at 240 nm using purified water in both sample and reference positions (1 × 1 × 4-cm fused silica cells, see section 4.5.2).

13. Add 4 ml of filtrate from the test-tube to a clean, dry cell, add 50 μl of concentrated ammonium hydroxide and mix using a plastic paddle. Check that the pH is about 10 (universal indicator paper).

14. Quickly measure the absorbance at 240 nm against a purified water blank (see section 4.5.2). If necessary, accurately dilute a portion of the extract with purified water to bring the reading on to the scale, and record the magnitude of the dilution. If a scanning spectro-photometer is available, scan in the region 200–450 nm.

15. Repeat the reading or scan after 5 minutes.

16. Add 0.1 ml of concentrated sulfuric acid to the cell, mix using the plastic paddle, and check that the pH is about 2 (universal indicator paper).

17. Repeat the reading (240 nm) or scan (200–450 nm).

Results

A number of compounds can interfere. Glutethimide is hydrolysed rapidly at alkaline pH values, so that the absorbance at 240 nm will markedly decrease after 5 minutes at pH 11 (step 15 above) if this compound is present. The presence of other compounds, such as methaqualone or phenazone (e.g., dichloralphenazone), can be revealed by scanning in the region 200–450 nm. Addition of 0.1 ml of aqueous sodium hydroxide (2 mol/l) to the ammoniacal extract (step 14 above) produces a further characteristic spectral change (Fig. 10) which can be useful in qualitative work.

To perform a quantitative measurement, measure the difference between absorbance at pH 10 and at pH 2, construct a calibration graph by analysis of the standard barbiturate solutions, and calculate the barbiturate concentration in the sample.

Alternatively, use the following formula:

((absorbance at pH10) − (absorbance at pH2)) × dilution factor (if any)
× 25 = barbiturate (mg/l)

Sample volumes of less than 5 ml may be used, but there will be a corresponding loss of sensitivity unless "micro"-volume fused silica spectrophotometer cells are available.

Sensitivity

Barbiturate, 2 mg/l.

Clinical interpretation

Barbiturates are very toxic in overdose and may cause peripheral vasodilation, hypotension, shock, hypoventilation, hypothermia, coma,

Fig. 10. Ultraviolet spectra of aqueous barbital sodium (50 mg/l) at different pH values

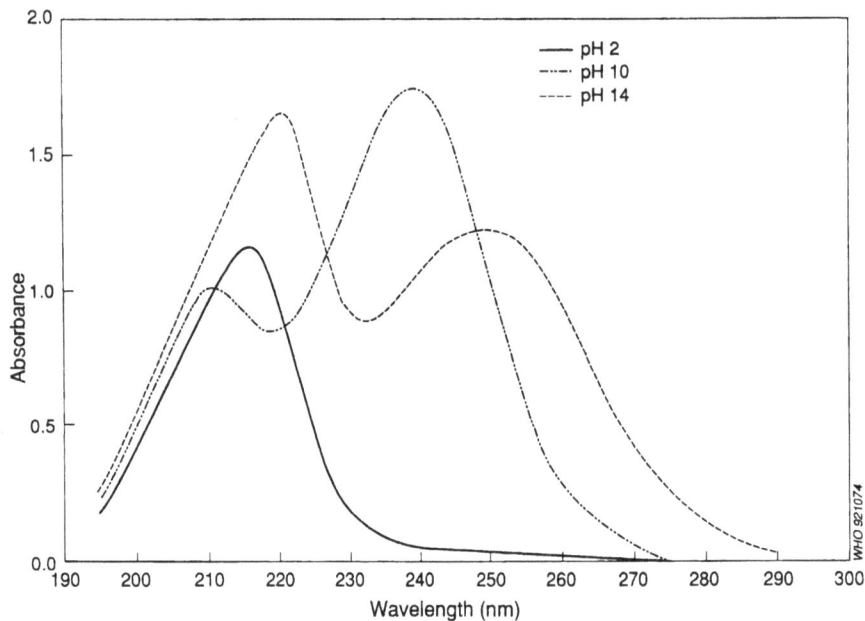

convulsions and acute renal failure. Death normally follows respiratory or cardiorespiratory arrest or respiratory complications.

Plasma barbiturate concentrations greater than 10 mg/l (50 mg/l barbital and phenobarbital) may be associated with serious toxicity. Repeated oral doses of activated charcoal and/or alkaline diuresis may be valuable in severe poisoning with barbital and phenobarbital. Charcoal haemoperfusion has been used to treat severe poisoning with short- and medium-acting barbiturates (see section 2.2.3).

6.10 Barium

The most important source of barium (Ba) is barium sulfate (barytes, $BaSO_4$) which is extremely insoluble in water. More soluble salts of barium, such as barium nitrate ($BaNO_3$) and barium chloride ($BaCl_2$), have a number of industrial uses and are relatively toxic. Barium sulfide (BaS) has been employed as a depilatory agent.

There is no simple method for the measurement of barium in biological specimens. However, the tests described below can be used to indicate the presence of barium salts in stomach contents or other samples that contain relatively high concentrations of the element.

The confirmatory test relies on the fact that lead sulfate is relatively soluble in dilute acetic acid but is precipitated in the presence of soluble barium salts, thus effectively enhancing the sensitivity of the reaction between barium and sulfate ions.

Qualitative test
Applicable to stomach contents and scene residues.

Reagents

1. Concentrated hydrochloric acid (relative density 1.18).
2. Platinum wire.

Method

1. Dip the end of the platinum wire in the concentrated acid.
2. Dip the moistened end of the wire into the test material.
3. Place the material in the hot part of the flame of a spirit lamp or microburner.

Results

A yellow-green flame indicates the presence of barium salts. Copper and thallium salts give a green flame in this test.

If large amounts of sodium salts are present, an orange/yellow coloration will obscure everything else.

Sensitivity

Barium, 50 mg/l.

Confirmatory test

Applicable to stomach contents and scene residues.

Reagents

1. Aqueous sulfuric acid (1 mol/l).
2. Aqueous lead acetate solution (100 g/l).
3. Aqueous acetic acid (50 ml/l).
4. Ammonium acetate (solid).

Method

1. Mix 2 ml of lead acetate solution and 2 ml of dilute sulfuric acid, and add sufficient ammonium acetate to dissolve the lead sulfate precipitate.
2. Add 0.1 ml of dilute acetic acid to 1 ml of sample, add 1 ml of the lead sulfo-acetate solution (from step 1), and vortex-mix for 5 seconds.
3. Centrifuge for 2 minutes and view the tube against a black background.

Results

A white turbidity or a white precipitate indicates the presence of barium. Calcium and strontium interfere in this test.

Sensitivity

Barium, 100 mg/l.

Clinical interpretation

The ingestion of soluble barium salts may produce gastroenteritis, ventricular fibrillation and muscular paralysis. Life-threatening hypokalaemia is an important feature of severe barium poisoning (see section 3.1.2).

6.11 Benzodiazepines

Most of these compounds have the general structure shown below:

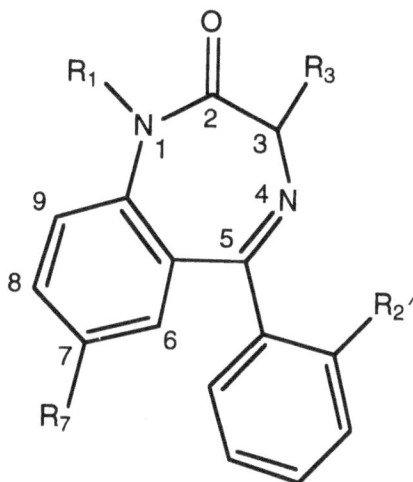

Some common benzodiazepines are listed in Table 19. Alprazolam, camazepam, clorazepate, flunitrazepam, ketazolam, loprazolam, lormetazepam, medazepam, midazolam, prazepam and triazolam are among the 60 or so members of this group.

Benzodiazepines are used as tranquillizers, and clobazam, clonazepam, and diazepam are also used as anticonvulsants. Temazepam especially has been abused, often together with other drugs. Most benzodiazepines are extensively metabolized and many members of this group are in fact metabolites of other compounds. Thus, diazepam gives nordazepam, oxazepam (3-hydroxynordazepam), and temazepam (3-hydroxydiazepam), which are excreted in urine as glucuronide or sulfate conjugates.

There is no reliable colour test for these compounds. However, on hydrolysis most benzodiazepines and their conjugates give rise to aminobenzophenones which can be extracted and analysed by thin-layer chromatography. Two different spray reagents are used to increase the discriminating power of the method, *p*-dimethylaminocinnamaldehyde and nitrous acid/*N*-(1-naphthyl)ethylenediamine (the Bratton-Marshall reaction).

Qualitative test

Applicable to urine, stomach contents and scene residues.

Table 19. Some common benzodiazepines

Compound	Chemical name	Relative molecular mass
Chlordiazepoxide	7-Chloro-2-methylamino-5-phenyl-3*H*-1,4-benzodiazepine 4-oxide	300
Clobazam	7-Chloro-1-methyl-5-phenyl-1*H*-1,5-benzodiazepin-2,4(3*H*,5*H*)-dione	301
Clonazepam	5-(2-Chlorophenyl)-1,3-dihydro-7-nitro-2*H*-1,4-benzodiazepin-2-one	316
Diazepam	7-Chloro-1,3-dihydro-1-methyl-5-phenyl-2*H*-1,4-benzodiazepin-2-one	285
Flurazepam	7-Chloro-1-(2-diethylaminoethyl)-5-(2-fluoro-phenyl)-1,3-dihydro-2*H*-1,4-benzodiazepin-2-one	388
Lorazepam	7-Chloro-5-(2-chlorophenyl)-1,3-dihydro-3-hydroxy-2,*H*-1,4-benzodiazepin-2-one	321
Nitrazepam	1,3-Dihydro-7-nitro-5-phenyl-2*H*-1,4-benzodiazepin-2-one	281
Oxazepam	7-Chloro-1,3-dihydro-3-hydroxy-5-phenyl-2*H*-1,4-benzodiazepin-2-one	287
Temazepam	7-Chloro-1,3-dihydro-3-hydroxy-1-methyl-5-phenyl-2*H*-1,4-benzodiazepin-2-one	301

Reagents

1. Concentrated hydrochloric acid (relative density 1.18).
2. Petroleum ether (40-60 °C boiling fraction).
3. Silica gel thin-layer chromatography plate (10 × 20 cm; 20 μm average particle size; see section 4.4.1).
4. Aqueous hydrochloric acid (1 mol/l).
5. Toluene:glacial acetic acid (97:3).
6. Aqueous *p*-dimethylaminocinnamaldehyde solution (5 g/l).
7. Aqueous trichloroacetic acid (500 g/l).
8. Aqueous sulfuric acid (500 ml/l).
9. Aqueous sodium nitrite solution (10 g/l, freshly prepared).
10. Aqueous ammonium sulfamate solution (50 g/l).
11. *N*-(1-Naphthyl)ethylenediamine hydrochloride (10 g/l) in acetone:water (4:1).

Standards

Flurazepam and nitrazepam, both at concentrations of 100 mg/l in dilute hydrochloric acid (1 mol/l).

Method

1. Mix 3 ml of concentrated hydrochloric acid and 10 ml of sample or standard in a 30-ml glass tube with a ground-glass stopper.
2. Place the unstoppered tube in a boiling water-bath **in a fume cupboard** for 30 minutes.
3. Cool, add 10 ml of petroleum ether, stopper the tube and rotary-mix for 10 minutes.
4. Centrifuge in a bench centrifuge for 5 minutes and transfer the upper, organic layer to a clean tube.
5. Evaporate the extract to dryness under a stream of compressed air or nitrogen at 60 °C.

Thin-layer chromatography

1. Reconstitute the extract in 100 μl of petroleum ether.
2. Divide the plate into four (two pairs of two columns), and spot two 25-μl portions of the sample and standard extracts on to each pair of columns (sample extracts first, see section 4.4.2)
3. Develop the chromatogram (10-cm run) using toluene:acetic acid (saturated tank, see section 4.4.3).
4. Remove the plate and allow to dry.

**Take care — all of the spray reagents used are toxic.
Spraying must be performed in a fume cupboard
or under an efficient fume hood.**

5. Spray one pair of columns (A) with *p*-dimethylaminocinnamaldehyde solution followed by trichloroacetic acid.
6. Spray the remaining pair of columns (B) with the following reagents, drying between each stage: sulfuric acid, sodium nitrite solution, ammonium sulfamate solution and naphthylethylenediamine solution.

Results

hR_f values and colour reactions of some common benzophenones are given in Table 20.

Interference from other hydrolysis products can be minimized by extracting the petroleum ether extract (step 4) with aqueous sodium hydroxide (2 mol/l) on a rotary mixer for 5 minutes. Subsequently, separate the phases by centrifugation for 5 minutes, and evaporate the petroleum ether extract to dryness as described above (step 5).

Interpretation of the results can be difficult since many compounds give methylaminochlorobenzophenone and/or aminochlorobenzophen-

Table 20. Thin-layer chromatography of aminobenzophenones: hR$_f$ values and colour reactions

Benzophenone	Derived from:	Origin	hR$_f$	Colour A^a	B^b
Methylamino-chloro-	Diazepam	Diazepam Ketazolam Medazepam	66	Pink	Purple
	Temazepam	Temazepam Diazepam Camazepam Medazepam Ketazolam			
Aminochloro-	Oxazepam	Oxazepam Diazepam Prazepam Medazepam Ketazolam Chlordiazepoxide Camazepam Temazepam Dipotassium clorazepate	40	Purple	Purple
	Chlordiazepoxide	Chlordiazepoxide			
	Desmethylchlor-diazepoxide	Chlordiazepoxide			
	Demoxepam Nordazepam	Chlordiazepoxide Diazepam Dipotassium clorazepate Ketazolam Prazepam Medazepam Chlordiazepoxide			
Aminodichloro-	Lorazepam	Lorazepam Lormetazepam	45	Purple	Purple
Aminochloro-fluoro-	Desalkyl-flurazepam	Flurazepam	31	Purple	Purple
Aminonitro-	Nitrazepam	Nitrazepam	34	Pink	Purple
Diamino-	7-Amino-nitrazepam	Nitrazepam	52	Purple	Blue
	7-Acetamido-nitrazepam	Nitrazepam			

Table 20 (contd.)

Benzophenone	Derived from:	Origin	hR$_f$	Colour	
				A^a	B^b
Aminonitro-chloro-	Clonazepam Loprazolam and metabolites	Clonazepam Loprazolam	34	Pink	Blue

^{a} Visualization reagent: *p*-dimethylaminocinnamaldehyde solution followed by trichloroacetic acid.

^{b} Visualization reagent: sulfuric acid followed by sodium nitrite solution, ammonium sulfamate solution and naphthylethylenediamine solution.

one on hydrolysis of urine. For example, it may not be possible to differentiate between temazepam or oxazepam and diazepam or nordazepam since these compounds give a similar pattern of benzophenones.

The following compounds do not themselves give benzophenones on hydrolysis: medazepam, triazolam, clobazam, norclobazam, and midazolam.

Sensitivity

Nordazepam (as aminochlorobenzophenone), 1 mg/l.

Clinical interpretation

Acute poisoning with benzodiazepines is common but, in adults, usually causes only drowsiness, confusion, ataxia, slurred speech, incoordination and sometimes coma. Respiratory depression is unusual in adults except with flurazepam. However, respiratory depression may occur if respiratory disease is already present, and in young children and the elderly. Benzodiazepines also have a synergistic respiratory depressant effect when taken with ethanol or other central nervous system depressants.

Treatment is normally symptomatic and supportive, although flumazenil may be used as a specific antagonist (see Table 4, p. 8). There is little need to measure plasma benzodiazepine concentrations in the management of acute poisoning.

6.12 Bismuth

Bismuth (Bi) has industrial uses in pigments and the production of alloys. In medicine, the main applications of bismuth salts, such as bismuth subsalicylate, are for the treatment of gastrointestinal problems like gastritis, peptic ulcer and diarrhoea. As with antimony, arsenic and mercury, bismuth can be detected using the Reinsch test.

Qualitative test

Applicable to urine, stomach contents and scene residues. Reinsch test —see antimony monograph (section 6.5)

Results

Staining on the copper can be interpreted as follows:

purple black — antimony
dull black — arsenic
shiny black — bismuth
silvery — mercury

Selenium and tellurium may also give dark deposits, while high concentrations of sulfur may give a speckled appearance to the copper.

An estimation of the concentration of bismuth in the sample can be made by comparison of the deposit on the copper with that obtained from a solution containing a known concentration of the element.

Sensitivity

Bismuth, about 2 mg/l.

Confirmatory test

Applicable to blackened copper from the test above.

Reagents

1. Aqueous potassium cyanide solution (100 g/l). **Take care when using concentrated cyanide solutions**.
2. Aqueous sodium sulfite solution (50 g/l, freshly prepared).
3. Aqueous nitric acid (3 mol/l).
4. Quinine/potassium iodide reagent. Dissolve 1 g of quinine sulfate in 100 ml of purified water containing 0.5 ml of concentrated nitric acid (relative density 1.42). Add 2 g of potassium iodide when the quinine has completely dissolved.

Method

1. Place the copper in potassium cyanide solution and allow to stand for 10 minutes.

2. Wash any undissolved stain with purified water and add 1 ml of sodium sulfite solution and 1 ml of dilute nitric acid.
3. Agitate frequently for 5 minutes and add 1 ml of purified water followed by 1 ml of quinine/potassium iodide reagent.

Results

Stains due to arsenic dissolve in potassium cyanide solution, while stains due to antimony and bismuth do not. However, bismuth slowly forms an orange/brown suspension with quinine/potassium iodide reagent.

Sensitivity

Bismuth, about 2 mg/l.

Clinical interpretation

Acute poisoning with bismuth may cause renal damage, encephalopathy and peripheral neuropathy. Neurotoxicity may also occur after chronic treatment with bismuth salts, but is reversible if medication is stopped.

6.13 Borates

Borates are found in household products as either boric acid (H_3BO_3) or borax (sodium borate, disodium tetraborate, $Na_2B_4O_7$), and are used in insecticides, fungicides, wood-preservatives, cleaning agents and water softeners. Weak solutions are used in eye-drops, eye-lotions, mouth washes, depilatory agents and other topical ointments. Small children are especially susceptible to borates and deaths have occurred after topical application of boric acid powder for nappy rash. Serious borate poisoning in adults is usually the result of improper use. The fatal dose of boric acid or sodium borate in an adult is 7–35 g.

Qualitative test

Applicable to stomach contents and scene residues.

Reagents

1. Turmeric (the spice) solution (10 g/l) in methanol.
2. Aqueous hydrochloric acid (1 mol/l).
3. Aqueous ammonium hydroxide (4 mol/l).

Method

1. Soak strips (1 × 5 cm) of filter-paper in turmeric solution and allow to dry at room temperature.

2. Add 1 ml of dilute hydrochloric acid to 1 ml of sample and soak a strip of turmeric paper in the solution.
3. Allow the paper to dry and then moisten with ammonium hydroxide solution.

Results

A brownish-red colour is obtained initially which intensifies as the paper dries. A change to green-black upon moistening with ammonium hydroxide indicates the presence of borates. Oxidizing agents (including bromates, chlorates, iodates and nitrites) interfere because they bleach turmeric.

Sensitivity

Borate, 50 mg/l.

Confirmatory test

Applicable to stomach contents and scene residues.

Reagent

Carminic acid (0.5 g/l) in concentrated sulfuric acid (relative density 1.83).

Method

1. Filter, if necessary, 5 ml of stomach contents into a 10-ml glass tube.
2. Add 0.5 ml of filtrate or scene residue to a clean tube and **slowly** add 0.5 ml of carminic acid solution down the side of the tube so that it forms a layer under the sample.

Results

A blue-violet ring at the junction of the two layers indicates the presence of borate. Strong oxidizing agents (including bromates, chlorates, iodates and nitrites) also give positive results in this test.

Sensitivity

Borate, 100 mg/l.

Quantitative assay

Applicable to plasma or serum (1 ml).

Reagents

1. Aqueous ammonium sulfate solution (40 g/l).
2. Concentrated sulfuric acid (relative density 1.83).
3. Carminic acid (0.2 g/l) in concentrated sulfuric acid.

Standards

Dissolve 0.210 g of boric acid in 100 ml of purified water (borate ion, 2.00 g/l) and dilute with blank serum to give standard solutions containing borate ion concentrations of 20, 50, 100 and 200 mg/l.

Method

1. Add 5 ml of ammonium sulfate solution to 1 ml of sample or standard, vortex-mix, and heat in a boiling water-bath for 15 minutes.
2. Centrifuge for 10 minutes and transfer the supernatant to a 10-ml volumetric flask.
3. Shake the precipitate with 2 ml of water, centrifuge as above and again transfer the supernatant to the flask.
4. Make up to 10.0 ml with purified water and mix for 5 seconds.
5. To 1 ml of the solution from the flask add 5 ml of concentrated sulfuric acid and mix thoroughly.
6. Add 5 ml of carminic acid solution, mix thoroughly and allow to stand for 10 minutes.
7. Read the absorbance at 600 nm against a serum blank (see section 4.5.2).

Results

Plot a graph of absorbance against borate concentration in the calibration solutions and calculate the borate concentration in the sample.

Sensitivity

Borate, 20 mg/l.

Clinical interpretation

Clinical features of borate poisoning include nausea, vomiting, diarrhoea, coma, convulsions and circulatory collapse. Haemodialysis or peritoneal dialysis may be indicated in severe cases. Normally, serum borate concentrations range up to 7 mg/l, but serious toxicity may occur at concentrations of 20–150 mg/l. Death may occur at concentrations ranging from 200 mg/l to 1500 mg/l.

6.14 Bromates

Bromates, such as sodium bromate ($NaBrO_3$), are used as ingredients in hair treatment (home perm) kits and are strong oxidizing agents. The diphenylamine test given below will detect other such compounds, notably chlorates, hypochlorites, iodates, nitrates and nitrites.

Qualitative test

Applicable to stomach contents and scene residues.

Reagent

Diphenylamine (10 g/l) in concentrated sulfuric acid (relative density 1.83).

Method

1. Filter, if necessary, 5 ml of stomach contents into a 10-ml glass tube.
2. Add 0.5 ml of filtrate or scene residue to a clean tube and **slowly** add 0.5 ml of diphenylamine solution down the side of the tube so that it forms a layer under the sample.

Results

A positive result is indicated by a strong blue colour which develops immediately at the junction of the two layers. A light blue colour will be given by most samples of stomach contents owing to the presence of organic material. Since all strong oxidizing agents are rapidly reduced in biological samples, the test should be performed as soon as possible after receipt of the sample.

Sensitivity

Bromate, 10 mg/l.

Confirmatory test

Applicable to urine, stomach contents and scene residues.

Reagents

1. Aqueous nitric acid (2 mol/l).
2. Aqueous silver nitrate solution (10 g/l).
3. Aqueous sodium nitrite solution (50 g/l, freshly prepared).
4. Concentrated ammonium hydroxide (relative density 0.88).

Method

1. To 1 ml of sample add 0.2 ml of dilute nitric acid and 0.2 ml of silver nitrate solution and mix for 5 seconds.
2. If a precipitate forms (owing to the presence of halides), centrifuge in a bench centrifuge for 1 minute and retain the clear supernatant.
3. Add more silver nitrate solution, drop by drop, to ensure the complete removal of any halide, and then add 0.2 ml of sodium nitrite solution.

4. If a precipitate forms add 0.2 ml of concentrated ammonium hydroxide.

Results

A cream precipitate sparingly soluble in ammonium hydroxide indicates the presence of bromate. Iodate reacts similarly to halides in this test (see step 3).

Sensitivity

Bromate, 10 mg/l.

Clinical interpretation

Acute bromate poisoning may cause nausea, vomiting, diarrhoea, abdominal pain, confusion, coma and convulsions. Methaemoglobin-aemia is often produced and this may be indicated by dark chocolate-coloured blood (see section 3.2.2). Blood methaemoglobin can be measured but is unstable, and the use of stored samples is unreliable. Treatment is symptomatic and supportive.

6.15 Bromides

Salts such as sodium bromide (NaBr) are sometimes still used as sedatives and anticonvulsants, and are also employed in photographic processing. Methyl bromide is used as a fumigant in ships' holds and grain silos, and is partly metabolized to bromide ion *in vivo*. Brominated sedatives such as carbromal also give rise to inorganic bromide when metabolized. The qualitative test given below serves to indicate the presence of inorganic bromide or iodide, and the appropriate confirmatory tests must then be used.

Qualitative test

Applicable to urine, stomach contents and scene residues.

Reagents

1. Aqueous nitric acid (2 mol/l).
2. Aqueous silver nitrate solution (10 g/l).
3. Concentrated ammonium hydroxide (relative density 0.88).

Method

1. Add 0.1 ml of nitric acid to 1 ml of clear test solution, mix for 5 seconds and add 0.1 ml of silver nitrate solution.

2. Centrifuge to isolate any significant precipitate, decant and treat with
   0.1 ml of concentrated ammonium hydroxide.

Results

A white precipitate soluble in ammonium hydroxide indicates chloride,
an off-white precipitate sparingly soluble in ammonium hydroxide
indicates bromide, and a creamy yellow, insoluble precipitate indicates
iodide.

This procedure can also be used to test for organobromine sedatives
such as carbromal in stomach contents and scene residues. First boil 1 ml
of the sample with 1 ml of aqueous sodium hydroxide (5 mol/l) for
5 minutes, cool and neutralize by slowly adding 3 ml of nitric acid
(2 mol/l). Then proceed with step 1 above.

Sensitivity

Bromide, 50 mg/l.

Confirmatory test

Applicable to urine, stomach contents and scene residues.

Reagents

1. Saturated fluorescein solution in aqueous acetic acid (600 ml/l).
2. Concentrated sulfuric acid (relative density 1.83).
3. Potassium permanganate (solid)

Method

1. Soak a strip of filter-paper in fluorescein solution.
2. Add about 50 mg of potassium permanganate to 2 ml of test solution
   in a 10-ml test-tube.
3. Add 0.2 ml of concentrated sulfuric acid and hold the fluorescein-
   impregnated filter-paper in the mouth of the tube.

Results

Bromide is oxidized to free bromine. This reacts with the yellow dye
fluorescein to give eosin (tetrabromofluorescein) which has a pink/red
colour.

Sensitivity

Bromide, 50 mg/l.

Quantitative assay

Applicable to plasma or serum (2 ml).

Reagents

1. Aqueous chloroauric acid. Dissolve 0.5 g of chloroauric acid (gold chloride, $HAuCl_4 \cdot xH_2O$) in 100 ml of purified water.
2. Aqueous trichloroacetic acid (200 g/l).

Standards

Dissolve 1.29 g of sodium bromide in 500 ml of purified water (bromide ion 2 g/l). Prepare serial dilutions in purified water containing bromide ion concentrations of 0.2, 0.4, 0.6, 0.8, 1.2 and 1.6 g/l.

Method

1. Add 6 ml of trichloroacetic acid solution to 2 ml of sample in a 10-ml test-tube, vortex-mix for 30 seconds and allow to stand for 15 minutes.
2. Centrifuge in a bench centrifuge for 5 minutes and filter the supernatant through phase-separating filter-paper into a clean tube.
3. Add 1 ml of chloroauric acid solution to 4 ml of the clear supernatant and vortex-mix for 5 seconds.
4. Record the absorbance at 440 nm against a purified water blank (see section 4.5.2).

Results

Construct a calibration graph of bromide concentration against absorbance by analysis of the standard bromide solutions, and calculate the concentration of bromide ion in the sample. The calibration is linear for concentrations from 25 mg/l to 2.5 g/l. This method is not reliable with specimens that may give turbid supernatants, e.g. postmortem samples.

Sensitivity

Bromide, 25 mg/l.

Clinical interpretation

Following acute overdosage, bromides may cause nausea, vomiting and diarrhoea, but absorption is poor and systemic toxicity is more usual after chronic ingestion or exposure. In such cases, fatigue, irritability, anorexia, abdominal pain, skin pigmentation, visual and auditory hallucinations, delirium, tremor, ataxia and coma may occur.

Normal serum bromide concentrations are less than 10 mg/l but, following administration of bromides in therapy, concentrations of up to 80 mg/l may be attained. Toxicity is usually associated with bromide concentrations greater than 500 mg/l. Treatment is normally symptomatic and supportive.

6.16 Cadmium

Cadmium (Cd) forms colourless salts with chemical properties similar to those of zinc compounds. Cadmium oxide and cadmium salts and alloys are used in products such as nickel–cadmium dry batteries, solder, paint and plastic pigments. Acute poisoning due to cadmium is extremely rare, but chronic toxicity has been noted after occupational exposure and in some instances after the diet or the water supply has been contaminated, as with *itai-itai* (ouch-ouch) disease in Japan.

There is no simple qualitative test for cadmium that can be performed on biological samples or scene residues.

Clinical interpretation

Chronic exposure to cadmium may lead to renal tubular damage and impaired lung function. Osteomalacia has also been observed in cases where the diet is deficient in calcium. Ingestion of cadmium salts causes abdominal pain, vomiting and diarrhoea, with facial oedema, hypotension, metabolic acidosis, depressed respiration, pulmonary oedema, oliguria and death in severe cases. Treatment is symptomatic and supportive, and may include chelation therapy.

6.17 Caffeine

Methyltheobromine, 7-methyltheophylline, 1,3,7-trimethylxanthine; $C_8H_{10}N_4O_2$; relative molecular mass, 194

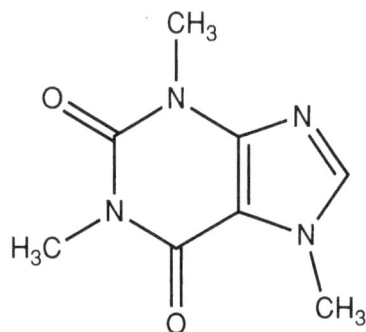

Caffeine is an alkaloid present in tea, coffee, cola and other beverages. A cup of coffee or tea may contain up to 100 mg of the drug. Caffeine is an ingredient of many proprietary stimulant preparations and is also used to treat neonatal apnoea. Metabolic reactions include *N*-demethylation and oxidation to uric acid derivatives. About 85% of an oral dose is excreted unchanged in urine. Caffeine is an important metabolite of theophylline in neonates, and in adults with impaired drug handling.

There is no simple qualitative test for caffeine, but this compound can be detected and identified by thin-layer chromatography of a basic solvent extract of urine, stomach contents or scene residues (see section 5.2.3). However, caffeine responds only to the acidified iodoplatinate visualization reagent, and sensitivity is poor.

Clinical interpretation

Acute overdosage with caffeine may cause palpitations, hypertension, diuresis, central nervous system stimulation, nausea, vomiting, marked hypokalaemia, metabolic acidosis and convulsions. Treatment is generally symptomatic and supportive.

6.18 Camphor

Bornan-2-one; $C_{10}H_{16}O$; relative molecular mass, 152

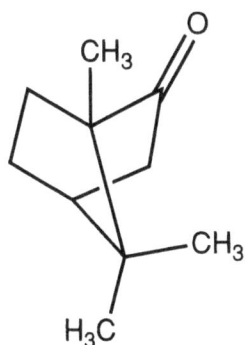

Camphor is a rubefacient and is also used in mothballs. It is obtained by distillation from the wood of *Cinnamomum camphora* or synthetically, and is metabolized by hydroxylation and excreted as glucuronides in urine. Camphor poisoning is usually due to ingestion of camphorated oil. The fatal dose in an adult may be as little as 4 g.

There is no simple qualitative test for this compound. However, camphor has a strong, distinctive smell and detection of this odour on the breath or in urine may aid the diagnosis.

Clinical interpretation

Ingestion of camphor may cause nausea, vomiting, headache, confusion, vertigo, excitement, hallucinations, tremor and dilated pupils. In severe cases, coma, convulsions and hepatorenal failure may ensure. Treatment is symptomatic and supportive.

6.19 Carbamate pesticides

These compounds have the general formula shown below. Substitution of sulfur for oxygen also occurs, but such compounds generally have low insecticidal activity. Some common carbamates are listed in Table 21.

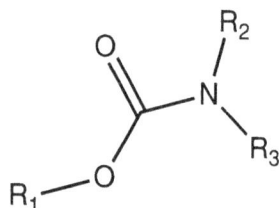

Table 21. Some carbamate pesticides

Compound	R_1	R_2	R_3	Relative molecular mass
Aldicarb	H	CH_3	$CH_3SC(CH_3)_2CH:N$	190
Carbaryl	H	CH_3	1-naphthyl	201
Methiocarb	H	CH_3	3,5-dimethyl-4-(methylthio)-phenyl	225
Pirimicarb	CH_3	CH_3	2-dimethylamino-5,6-dimethylpyrimidin-4-yl	238
Promecarb	H	CH_3	3-isopropyl-5-methylphenyl	207
Propoxur	H	CH_3	2-isopropoxyphenyl	209

Carbamates are widely used as insecticides, herbicides and fungicides. Carbamate insecticides inhibit acetylcholinesterase and thus evidence of exposure to such compounds can be obtained by measuring cholinesterase activity (see sections 3.1.5 and 6.30). Herbicide and fungicide carbamates, such as the dithiocarbamates, do not inhibit cholinesterase to any significant degree and are relatively nontoxic in humans. The test described here is based on a general reaction of carbamates with furfuraldehyde in the presence of hydrogen chloride.

Qualitative test

Applicable to stomach contents and scene residues.

Reagents

1. Aqueous hydrochloric acid (2 mol/l).
2. Furfuraldehyde solution (100 ml/l) in methanol, freshly prepared.
3. Concentrated hydrochloric acid (relative density 1.18).

Method:

1. Acidify 1 ml of sample with 0.5 ml of dilute hydrochloric acid and extract with 4 ml of chloroform on a rotary mixer for 5 minutes.
2. Centrifuge in a bench centrifuge for 5 minutes, discard the upper, aqueous layer and filter the chloroform extract through phase-separating filter-paper into a clean tube.
3. Evaporate the extract to dryness under a stream of compressed air or nitrogen at 40 °C.
4. Dissolve the residue in 0.1 ml of methanol, apply a spot of the solution to filter-paper and allow to dry.
5. Apply 0.1 ml of furfuraldehyde solution to the spot, allow to dry and expose the paper to concentrated hydrochloric acid fumes for 5 minutes **in a fume cupboard**.

Results

Carbamates give a black spot. Meprobamate and other non-pesticide carbamates interfere in this test.

Sensitivity

Carbamate, 100 mg/l.

Clinical interpretation

Exposure to carbamates may cause anorexia, abdominal pain, nausea, vomiting, diarrhoea, lacrimation, increased salivation, sweating, anxiety, ataxia and acute pulmonary oedema. Antidotal therapy with atropine may be indicated, but pralidoxime should not be used.

6.20 Carbamazepine

5*H*-Dibenz[*b,f*]azepine-5-carboxamide; $C_{15}H_{12}N_2O$; relative molecular mass, 236

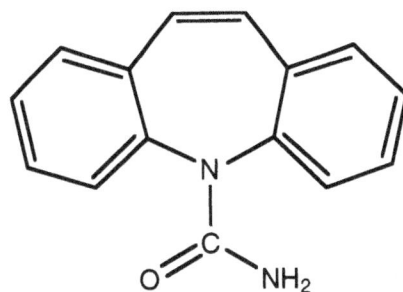

Carbamazepine is widely used as an anticonvulsant. Metabolic reactions include epoxidation to give carbamazepine-10,11-epoxide (which is pharmacologically active), diol formation, hydroxylation and conjugation. Less than 10% of a dose is excreted in urine as the parent compound. The estimated minimum lethal dose in an adult is 5 g.

Qualitative test

Applicable to stomach contents and scene residues.

Reagents

1. Aqueous hydrochloric acid (2 mol/l).
2. Sodium hypobromite reagent. Dissolve 0.5 ml of elemental bromine carefully and with cooling in 5 ml of aqueous sodium hydroxide solution (400 g/l). Prepare freshly.

Method

1. Add 1 ml of dilute hydrochloric acid to 5 ml of sample and 5 ml of chloroform, vortex-mix for 1 minute and centrifuge in a bench centrifuge for 5 minutes.
2. After discarding the upper, aqueous layer, add 1 ml of the chloroform extract to 0.2 ml of sodium hypobromite reagent in a clean tube and vortex-mix for 30 seconds.

Results

A blue-violet colour in the chloroform layer indicates the presence of carbamazepine. This compound and its metabolites can also be detected by thin-layer chromatography of an acidic extract of urine (see section 5.2.3).

Sensitivity

Carbamazepine, 250 mg/l.

Clinical interpretation

Carbamazepine poisoning may cause headache, dry mouth, abdominal discomfort, diarrhoea, constipation, ataxia, nystagmus, diplopia, hypotension, coma, convulsions and respiratory depression. Treatment is generally symptomatic and supportive.

6.21 Carbon disulfide

Carbon disulfide (CS_2) is used as a synthetic intermediate, a solvent (especially in viscose rayon manufacture), a grain and soil fumigant, an insecticide, a corrosion inhibitor and in degreasing. Some 50–90% of an ingested dose of carbon disulfide is metabolized and excreted in urine as inorganic sulfate, thiourea, 2-mercapto-2-thiazolin-5-one and 2-thio-thiazolidine-4-carboxylic acid (TTCA). Carbon disulfide has a particularly pungent smell. The ingestion of 15 ml may prove fatal in an adult.

There is no simple method for the detection of carbon disulfide in biological specimens other than by smell. However, the method given below can be used to assess exposure and relies on the fact that TTCA catalyses the decolorization of a solution of iodine by sodium azide.

Qualitative test

Applicable to urine.

Reagents

1. Iodine-azide reagent. Dissolve 3 g of sodium azide in 25 ml of purified water, add 50 ml of an aqueous solution containing iodine (24.5 g/l) and potassium iodide (50 g/l), and dilute to 100 ml.
2. Aqueous sodium dihydrogen orthophosphate (110 g/l).

Method

1. Add 0.2 ml of sodium dihydrogen orthophosphate solution to 1.0 ml of test urine and to 1.0 ml of blank urine in separate test-tubes.
2. Vortex-mix for 2 seconds, add 20 μl of iodine-azide reagent to each tube and again vortex-mix for 2 seconds.

Results

The yellow-brown colour (of iodine) is decolorized within 30 seconds in the presence of TTCA at room temperature. It is especially important to analyse the blank urine as well as the test urine in this instance, since urine itself often has a yellow-brown colour.

Sensitivity

TTCA, 10 mg/l.

Clinical interpretation

Carbon disulfide is an excellent solvent for fat, and dermal contact can cause reddening, burning, cracking and peeling of the skin. Acute poisoning from either ingestion or inhalation may give rise to irritation of mucous membranes, blurred vision, headache, nausea, vomiting, coma, convulsions and cardiorespiratory arrest.

Following chronic exposure, peripheral neuropathy, fatigue, sleep disturbance, anorexia, weight loss, depression, intellectual impairment, diabetes mellitus and ischaemic heart disease may occur. Treatment is generally symptomatic and supportive.

6.22 Carbon monoxide

Carbon monoxide (CO) is an important constituent of coal gas, but is not present in natural gas. Nowadays, common sources of carbon monoxide are automobile exhaust fumes, improperly maintained or ventilated gas or fuel oil heating systems, and smoke from all types of fires. Carbon monoxide is also produced *in vivo* from the metabolism of dichloromethane.

Carbon monoxide is highly poisonous and combines with haemoglobin and other haem proteins such as cytochrome oxidase, thereby limiting the oxygen supply to tissue and inhibiting cellular respiration. The affinity of carbon monoxide for haemoglobin is about 200 times that of oxygen. Thus, severe acute or acute-on-chronic poisoning can occur when relatively small quantities of carbon monoxide are present in the inspired air.

The qualitative test described below is relatively insensitive and is useful only in the diagnosis of acute carbon monoxide poisoning. If a positive result is obtained then either the blood carboxyhaemoglobin (HbCO) or the breath carbon monoxide concentration should be measured without delay. The quantitative method for determining blood HbCO described below relies on the fact that both oxygenated haemoglobin and methaemoglobin (oxidized haemoglobin) can be reduced by sodium dithionite while HbCO is largely unaffected.

Qualitative test

Applicable to whole blood treated with heparin, edetic acid or fluoride/oxalate.

Reagent

Aqueous ammonium hydroxide (0.01 mol/l).

Method

Add 0.1 ml of blood to 2 ml of ammonium hydroxide solution and vortex-mix for 5 seconds.

Results

A pink tint in comparison with the colour obtained from a normal blood specimen suggests the presence of carboxyhaemoglobin. Cyanide may give a similar tint, but acute cyanide poisoning is generally much less common than carbon monoxide poisoning.

Sensitivity

HbCO, 20%.

Quantitative assay

Applicable to whole blood treated with heparin, edetic acid or fluoride/oxalate.

Reagents

1. Aqueous ammonium hydroxide (1 ml/l).
2. Sodium dithionite (solid, stored in a desiccator).
3. A supply of pure carbon monoxide or carbon monoxide/nitrogen.
4. A supply of oxygen or compressed air.

Method

1. Add 0.2 ml of blood to 25 ml of ammonium hydroxide solution and mix.
2. Take three approximately equal portions: x, y and z. Keep portion x in a stoppered tube while the following procedures are performed:
   (*a*) Saturate portion y with carbon monoxide (to give 100% HbCO) by bubbling the gas through the solution for 5–10 minutes. Take care to minimize frothing.
   (*b*) Saturate portion z with oxygen by bubbling pure oxygen or compressed air through the solution for at least 10 minutes to remove all bound carbon monoxide (to give 0% HbCO). Again, take care to minimize frothing.
3. Add a small amount (about 20 mg) of sodium dithionite to each test solution (x, y and z) and also to 10 ml of ammonium hydroxide solution and mix well.
4. Measure the absorbances of solutions x, y and z against the dithionite-treated ammonium hydroxide solution at 540 nm and 579 nm.

Results

The percentage carboxyhaemoglobin saturation (% HbCO) can be calculated from the equation:

$$\%\text{HbCO} = \frac{(A_{540}/A_{579}\text{solution x}) - (A_{540}/A_{579}\text{solution z})}{(A_{540}/A_{579}\text{solution y}) - (A_{540}/A_{579}\text{solution z})} \times 100$$

Approximate normal values are:

$(A_{540}/A_{579}$ solution y$) = 1.5$, corresponding to 100% HbCO

$(A_{540}/A_{579}$ solution z$) = 1.1$, corresponding to 0% HbCO.

Note that the haemoglobin content of blood varies from person to person, and thus the volume of diluent used may need to be altered. A dilution giving a maximum absorbance of about 1 absorbance unit at 540 nm is ideal.

It is important to use sodium dithionite that has been freshly obtained or stored in a sealed container in a desiccator, since this compound is inactivated by prolonged contact with moist air.

This method is unreliable in the presence of other pigments such as methaemoglobin (indicated by a relatively high absorbance in the region 580–600 nm, see Fig. 11). Lipaemic blood specimens may give turbid suspensions which also give unreliable results.

The measurements are performed at the point of maximum difference of absorbance (540 nm, λ_{max} HbCO) and the point of equal absorbance

Fig. 11. Spectra obtained using a blood sample from a patient poisoned with carbon monoxide (A), 100% HbCO (B), and 0% HbCO (reduced haemoglobin) (C)

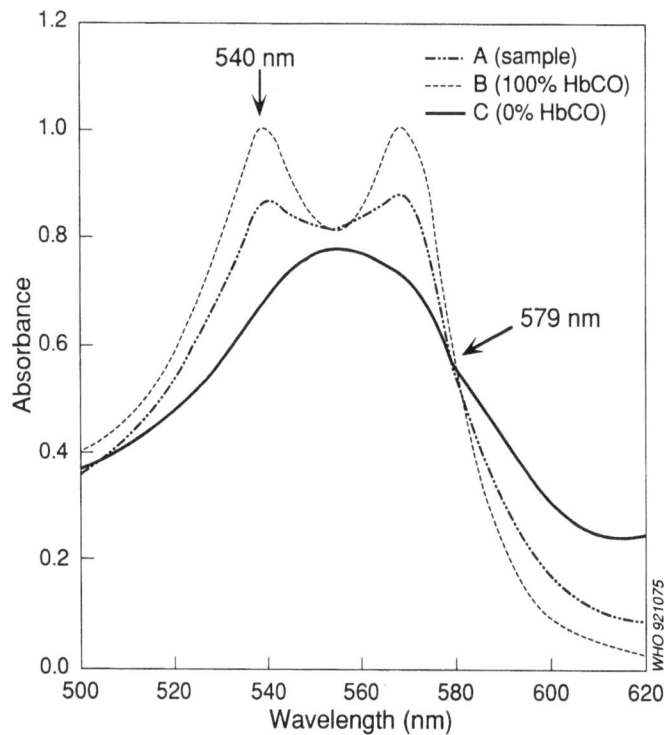

(579 nm, isobestic point). The reading at 579 nm is taken on a very steep slope (Fig. 11), and the wavelength is critical. Spectrophotometers with a relatively broad band-pass (4–5 nm) should not be used, since it will be impossible to perform the measurement with the accuracy required. Even if an instrument with a narrow band-pass is available, it is important to ensure that it is accurately calibrated, although the effect of minor variations can be minimized by using the following procedure:

1. Measure the absorbance of solution z (0% HbCO) against the dithionite-treated ammonium hydroxide solution at 540 nm. If the ratio (A_{540}/A_{579}) for 0% HbCO is assumed to be 1.1, the absorbance of this solution at 579 nm can be calculated.

2. Adjust the wavelength setting of the instrument to give this reading if not already attained at 579 nm. Alternatively, the spectra from the three solutions can be recorded using a scanning spectrophotometer, if available, and the measurements performed directly. Examples of the spectra that should be obtained are given in Figure 11. The presence of the twin absorption peaks ("rabbit's ears") is a useful qualitative feature.

Sensitivity

HbCO, approximately 10%.

Clinical interpretation

Features of acute carbon monoxide poisoning include headache, nausea, vomiting, haematemesis, hyperventilation, cardiac arrhythmias, pulmonary oedema, coma and acute renal failure. Cyanosis is commonly absent, so that skin and mucosae remain pink even in the presence of severe tissue hypoxia. Death often ensues from respiratory failure. Late neuropsychiatric sequelae are an increasingly recognized complication.

Treatment consists of removal from the contaminated atmosphere and administration of 100% oxygen via a well-fitting face-mask. Hyperbaric oxygen may be indicated in certain cases, and is especially effective in preventing the development of late sequelae, but facilities where this can be given are rare.

Once the patient is removed from the contaminated atmosphere, carboxyhaemoglobin is dissociated rapidly, especially if oxygen is administered in treatment. HbCO measurements are therefore often unhelpful as an indication of the severity of poisoning except in forensic toxicology. A simple guide to the interpretation of blood HbCO results is given in Table 22.

Table 22. Interpretation of blood carboxyhaemoglobin (HbCO) results

HbCO saturation (%)	Associated with:
3–8	Cigarette smokers
< 15	Heavy smokers (30–50 cigarettes per day)
20	Danger to heart disease patients
20–50	Progressive loss of mental and physical coordination resembling ethanol intoxication
> 50	Coma, convulsions, cardiorespiratory arrest, death

6.23 Carbon tetrachloride

Tetrachloromethane; CCl_4; relative molecular mass, 154

Carbon tetrachloride was widely used as a dry-cleaning and degreasing agent and in fire extinguishers. However, as with chloroform, exposure to carbon tetrachloride frequently gives rise to hepatorenal damage and nowadays usage is largely restricted to fumigation of grain and industrial applications.

Massive exposure to carbon tetrachloride may be detectable in urine using the Fujiwara test, possibly because chloroform is a minor metabolite or contaminant; carbon tetrachloride itself does not react in this test.

Qualitative test

Applicable to urine. Fujiwara test. **This test must be performed in a fume cupboard.**

Reagents

1. Aqueous sodium hydroxide solution (5 mol/l, i.e., 200 g/l).
2. Aqueous trichloroacetic acid (10 mg/l).

Method

1. To separate 10-ml tubes add 1-ml portions of:
   (a) test urine;
   (b) purified water; and
   (c) trichloroacetic acid solution.
2. Add 1 ml of sodium hydroxide solution and 1 ml of pyridine to each tube, mix gently and fit with a loose stopper.
3. Heat in a boiling water-bath for 2 minutes.

Results

An intense red/purple colour in the upper, pyridine layer indicates the presence of trichloro compounds. The blank analysis excludes contamination with compounds such as chloroform from the laboratory atmosphere. Compounds such as chloral hydrate, dichloralphenazone and trichloroethylene, which are extensively metabolized to trichloroacetic acid, give strong positive results in this test.

Sensitivity

Trichloroacetate, 1 mg/l.

Clinical interpretation

Acute poisoning with carbon tetrachloride is rare. Clinical features include ataxia, nausea, vomiting, coma, convulsions, respiratory depression and cardiac arrhythmias. Hepatic and renal damage commonly occur. Treatment is symptomatic and supportive, although acetylcysteine may protect against liver and kidney damage.

6.24 Chloral hydrate

Chloral; 2,2,2-trichloroethane-1,1-diol; $C_2H_3O_2Cl_3$; relative molecular mass, 165

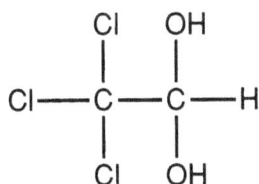

Chloral hydrate is a mild sedative and hypnotic agent. The pharmacological activity of chloral, and of the related compound dichloralphenazone, is thought to derive largely from a metabolite, 2,2,2-trichloroethanol, which is in turn metabolized to trichloroacetic acid. This latter compound can be detected in urine using the Fujiwara test.

Qualitative test

Applicable to urine. Fujiwara test — see carbon tetrachloride monograph (section 6.23). **This test must be performed in a fume cupboard.**

Results

An intense red/purple colour in the upper, pyridine layer indicates the presence of trichloro compounds. The blank (purified water) analysis excludes contamination with compounds such as chloroform from the laboratory atmosphere. Other trichloro compounds react in this test, but trichloroacetic acid is by far the most common compound encountered.

This test is very sensitive and will detect a therapeutic dose of chloral hydrate 12–24 hours after ingestion. However, other compounds, notably the solvent trichloroethylene, also give rise to trichloroacetic acid *in vivo* and caution must be exercised in reporting results.

Sensitivity

Trichloroacetate, 1 mg/l.

Clinical interpretation

Acute poisoning with chloral hydrate can cause vomiting, excitement, ataxia, confusion, drowsiness, stupor, hypotension, coma, cardiac arrhythmias, respiratory depression and pulmonary oedema. Treatment is normally symptomatic and supportive.

6.25 Chloralose

α-Chloralose; (*R*)-1,2-*O*-(2,2,2-trichloroethylidene)-α-D-glucofuranose; $C_8H_{11}Cl_3O_6$; relative molecular mass, 310

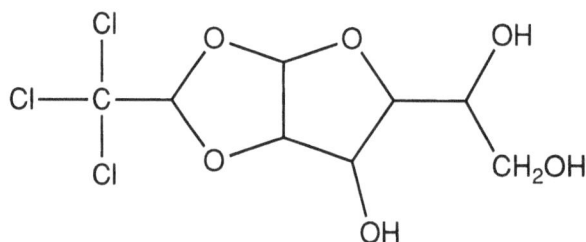

Chloralose is a hypnotic drug and has been used as a surgical anaesthetic in laboratory animals. It is also used as a bird repellent on seed grain and as a rodenticide, especially against mice, in cooler climates. The dose associated with toxicity in adults is about 1 g.

Chloralose may be oxidized with periodic acid to trichloroacetic acid, which can be detected using the Fujiwara test as for carbon tetrachloride. It was thought that chloralose undergoes hydrolysis *in vivo*, and that urine from patients who had ingested chloralose would give a positive reaction without periodate oxidation. However, recent work suggests that this is not the case.

Qualitative test

Applicable to plasma or serum, urine, stomach contents and scene residues. **This test must be performed in a fume cupboard.**

Reagents

1. Periodic acid reagent. Mix 3 g of sodium periodate and 3 ml of aqueous sulfuric acid (0.5 mol/l) and dilute to 100 ml with water.
2. Aqueous sodium hydroxide solution (5 mol/l, i.e., 200 g/l).
3. Aqueous trichloroacetic acid (10 mg/l).

Method

1. Add 1 ml of periodic acid reagent to 1 ml of test solution (or a portion of a solid residue extracted with 1 ml of water) in a 10-ml glass test-tube.
2. Mix and allow to stand for 5 minutes.
3. To separate 10-ml tubes add 2-ml portions of:
   (*a*) test solution;
   (*b*) purified water;
   (*c*) trichloroacetic acid solution.
4. Add 1 ml of sodium hydroxide solution and 1 ml of pyridine to all four tubes, mix gently and fit with a loose stopper.
5. Heat in a boiling water-bath for 2 minutes.

Results

An intense red/purple colour in the upper, pyridine layer of the periodate-treated tube indicates the presence of chloralose. The sample analysis without periodate is to exclude the presence of compounds, such as chloral hydrate, that give rise to trichloroacetic acid *in vivo*. The blank analysis excludes contamination with chloroform from the laboratory atmosphere.

Sensitivity

Trichloroacetate, 1 mg/l.

Clinical interpretation

Ingestion of chloralose may cause drowsiness, hypotonia and coma. Treatment is generally symptomatic and supportive.

6.26 Chlorates

Sodium chlorate ($NaClO_3$) is used as a weedkiller and in matches and fireworks. Chlorates are also used in small amounts in throat gargles and toothpastes. In an adult, serious poisoning may follow the ingestion of 15 g of sodium chlorate. Chlorates are strong oxidizing agents, and the test given below will also detect compounds with similar properties, such as bromates, hypochlorites, iodates, nitrates and nitrites.

Qualitative test

Applicable to stomach contents and scene residues.

Reagent

Diphenylamine (10 g/l) in concentrated sulfuric acid (relative density 1.83).

Method

1. Filter 5 ml of stomach contents into a 10-ml glass tube.
2. Add 0.5 ml of filtrate or scene residue to a clean tube and **slowly** add 0.5 ml of diphenylamine solution down the side of the tube so that it forms a layer under the sample.

Results

A true positive is indicated by a strong blue colour which develops immediately at the junction of the two layers. A light blue colour will be given by most samples of stomach contents owing to the presence of organic material. Since all strong oxidizing agents are reduced rapidly in biological samples, the test should be performed as soon as possible after receipt of the sample.

Sensitivity

Chlorate, 10 mg/l.

Confirmatory test

Applicable to stomach contents and scene residues.

Reagents

1. Manganous sulfate reagent. Mix saturated aqueous manganous sulfate with *o*-phosphoric acid (1:1).
2. Diphenylcarbazide (10 g/l) in methanol.

Method

1. To 0.1 ml of test solution add 0.2 ml of manganous sulfate reagent and warm briefly over a spirit lamp or microburner.
2. Cool and add 0.1 ml of diphenylcarbazide solution.

Results

A purple/violet colour, which is intensified after cooling and adding diphenylcarbazide, indicates chlorate.

Persulfates and periodates give a similar reaction; persulfates can be eliminated by evaporating the test solution with 0.1 ml of concentrated sulfuric acid (relative density 1.83) and 0.1 ml of aqueous silver nitrate (10 g/l).

Sensitivity

Chlorate, 100 mg/l.

Clinical interpretation

Acute poisoning with chlorates may cause nausea, vomiting, diarrhoea, abdominal pain, confusion, coma and convulsions. Methaemoglobin-aemia is often produced and this may be indicated by dark chocolate-coloured blood (see section 3.2.2). Blood methaemoglobin can be measured but is unstable, and the use of stored samples is unreliable. Treatment is symptomatic and supportive.

6.27 Chloroform

Trichloromethane; $CHCl_3$; relative molecular mass, 119

Chloroform was used as an anaesthetic and general solvent, but is relatively toxic since it is partly metabolized to phosgene ($COCl_2$) which is a potent hepatorenal toxin.

Chloroform can be detected readily using the Fujiwara test. However, this test will also detect ingestion or exposure to compounds that are extensively metabolized to trichloroacetic acid, such as chloral hydrate, dichloralphenazone and trichloroethylene.

Qualitative test

Applicable to urine. Fujiwara test — see carbon tetrachloride monograph (section 6.23). **This test must be performed in a fume cupboard.**

Results

An intense red/purple colour in the upper, pyridine layer indicates the presence of trichloro compounds. The blank analysis excludes contamination with compounds such as chloroform from the laboratory atmosphere. Trichloroacetic acid is by far the most common compound encountered in this test.

Sensitivity

Trichloroacetate, 1 mg/l.

Clinical interpretation

Acute poisoning with chloroform is rare. Clinical features include ataxia, nausea, vomiting, coma, convulsions, respiratory depression, cardiac arrhythmias and hepatorenal damage. Treatment is symptomatic and supportive. Acetylcysteine may protect against hepatorenal damage (see Table 4, p. 8).

6.28 Chlorophenoxy herbicides

These compounds have the general formula shown below. Some common chlorophenoxy herbicides are listed in Table 23.

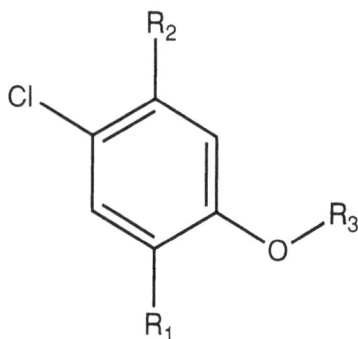

Table 23. Some chlorophenoxy herbicides

Compound	Chemical name	R_1	R_2	R_3	Relative molecular mass
2,4-D	2,4-Dichlorophenoxyacetic acid	Cl	H	CH_2COOH	221
2,4-DP (dichlorprop)	2-(2,4-Dichlorophenoxy)-propionic acid	Cl	H	$CH(CH_3)COOH$	235
MCPA	4-Chloro-2-methylphenoxy-acetic acid	CH_3	H	CH_2COOH	201
MCPP (mecoprop)	2-(4-Chloro-2-methylphenoxy)-propionic acid	CH_3	H	$CH(CH_3)COOH$	215
2,4,5-T	2,4,5-Trichlorophenoxy-acetic acid	Cl	Cl	CH_2COOH	256
2,4,5-TP (fenoprop)	2-(2,4,5-Trichlorophenoxy)-propionic acid	Cl	Cl	$CH(CH_3)COOH$	270

2,4-D (not to be confused with DNOC, i.e. dinitro-*o*-cresol, see section 6.42) and related compounds are used to control broad-leaved weeds in lawns and in cereal crops and, at higher application rates, for total vegetation control. They are frequently encountered as mixtures, both with other members of the group and with other pesticides.

Qualitative test

Applicable to stomach contents and scene residues.

Reagents

1. Aqueous hydrochloric acid (1 mol/l).
2. Sodium nitrite (100 g/l) in concentrated sulfuric acid (relative density 1.83), freshly prepared. **Take care — brown nitrogen dioxide fumes may be evolved**.
3. Chromotropic acid (2,5-dihydroxynaphthalene-2,7-disulfonic acid) (2 g/l) in concentrated sulfuric acid (relative density 1.83).

Method

1. Add 1 ml of dilute hydrochloric acid to 10 ml of sample, and extract with 20 ml of toluene on a rotary mixer for 5 minutes.
2. Centrifuge for 5 minutes, remove the upper, toluene layer, and extract the residue with a second 20-ml portion of toluene.
3. Combine the toluene extracts and evaporate to dryness under a stream of compressed air or nitrogen in a water-bath at 60 °C.
4. Dissolve the residue in 0.2 ml of concentrated sulfuric acid and divide between two wells of a porcelain spotting tile.
5. Add 0.1 ml of sodium nitrite solution to one well and 0.1 ml of chromotropic acid solution to the other.
6. Heat the tile in a beaker over a boiling water-bath or on a hot plate at 80 °C.

Results

The colours given by some common chlorophenoxy compounds are given in Table 24. These tests are not specific and can only be used to indicate the presence of chlorophenoxy compounds.

Sensitivity

Chlorophenoxy compounds, 500 mg/l.

Clinical interpretation

Absorption of chlorophenoxy herbicides may lead to vomiting, diarrhoea, areflexia, muscle weakness, pulmonary oedema and coma, with

Table 24. Colour reactions of some chlorophenoxy compounds

Compound[a]	With sodium nitrite	With chromotropic acid
2,4-D	Brown	Purple
2,4,-DP	Dark brown	Light purple
MCPA	Light brown	Light purple
MCPP	Light brown	Purple
2,4,5-T	No reaction	Purple
2,4,5-TP	No reaction	Light pink/purple

[a] For full chemical names see Table 23.

death in severe cases. Alkalinization may increase the renal excretion of 2,4-D and other chlorophenoxy compounds, and also protect against systemic toxicity (see section 2.2.3).

6.29 Chloroquine

7-Chloro-4-(4-diethylamino-1-methylbutylamino)quinoline; $C_{18}H_{26}ClN_3$; relative molecular mass, 320

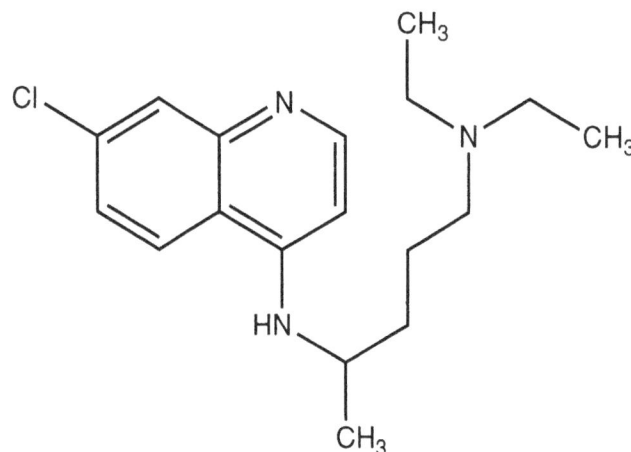

Chloroquine is a derivative of 4-aminoquinoline and is commonly used to treat malaria. Chloroquine has a long half-life in the body (25–60 days) and several metabolic products are formed, initially by *N*-dealkylation and deamination. As little as 1 g of chloroquine may cause death in a young child, and fatalities in adults have occurred after the ingestion of between 3 and 44 g.

There is no simple test for chloroquine in biological fluids, but this compound and its metabolites can be detected by thin-layer chromatography of a basic extract of urine (see section 5.2.3). Like quinine, chloroquine fluoresces under ultraviolet light (254 nm and 366 nm), and this provides an additional feature to aid identification.

Clinical interpretation

Acute chloroquine poisoning can develop within 30 minutes of ingestion. Clinical features include nausea, vomiting, abdominal pain, diarrhoea, tinnitus, blurred vision, dizziness, agitation, hypotension, coma, convulsions and respiratory depression. Sudden cardiorespiratory arrest may occur in severe cases. Treatment is generally symptomatic and supportive, but the specific combination of diazepam and epinephrine has proved particularly effective.

6.30 Cholinesterase activity

Many insecticides, such as carbamate and organophosphorus compounds, interfere with nerve transmission by inhibiting acetylcholinesterase. Semi-quantitative measurement of plasma cholinesterase activity provides a simple method of assessing exposure to these compounds (see section 3.1.5).

Qualitative test

Applicable to plasma or serum.

Reagents

1. Dithiobisnitrobenzoate reagent. 5,5'-Dithiobis(2-nitrobenzoic acid) (0.2 g/l) in sodium dihydrogen orthophosphate buffer (0.1 mol/l, pH 7.4).
2. Aqueous acetylthiocholine iodide solution (5 g/l).
3. Aqueous pralidoxime chloride solution (200 g/l).
4. Plasma or serum from an unexposed individual (control plasma).

Method

1. Add 2.0 ml of dithiobisnitrobenzoate reagent and 1.0 ml of acetylthiocholine iodide solution to each of three 10-ml test-tubes.
2. Add 20 µl of control plasma to one tube and 20 µl of test plasma to a second.
3. Add 20 µl of pralidoxime solution and 20 µl of test plasma to the third tube.
4. Vortex-mix the contents of all three tubes and allow to stand at room temperature for 2 minutes.

Results

The presence of an acetylcholinesterase inhibitor is indicated if the yellow colour in the control tube is deeper than in the test tube. If the colour in the tube containing pralidoxime is similar to that in the control tube, this provides further confirmation that an inhibitor of acetylcholinesterase is present in the sample (see section 3.1.5).

Clinical interpretation

Exposure to organophosphorus pesticides may cause bronchorrhoea, respiratory distress, excessive salivation, nausea, muscle weakness and eventually paralysis. Treatment is supportive, but should also include the administration of atropine and pralidoxime.

Exposure to carbamate pesticides may cause anorexia, abdominal pain, nausea, vomiting, diarrhoea, lacrimation, increased salivation, sweating, anxiety, ataxia and acute pulmonary oedema. Antidotal therapy with atropine may be indicated, but pralidoxime should not be used.

6.31 Clomethiazole

Chlormethiazole; 5-(2-chloroethyl)-4-methylthiazole; C_6H_8ClNS; relative molecular mass, 162

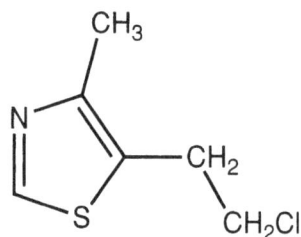

Clomethiazole is used as a hypnotic in elderly patients, as an anticonvulsant, and in the treatment of alcohol dependence and drug withdrawal. Less than 5% of an oral dose is excreted unchanged in urine, and a large number of metabolites have been identified. Clomethiazole has a characteristic smell on the breath and in stomach contents.

There is no simple qualitative test for clomethiazole, but this compound and its metabolites can be detected and identified by thin-layer chromatography of a basic solvent extract of urine (see section 5.2.3).

Clinical interpretation

Acute poisoning with clomethiazole may cause sneezing, increased salivation, conjunctival irritation, hypotension, hypothermia, coma and respiratory depression. Ethanol potentiates the depressant effects of clomethiazole on the central nervous system, and these compounds are often encountered together in fatal cases. Treatment is symptomatic and supportive.

6.32 Cocaine

Methyl benzoylecgonine; (1*R*,2*R*,3*s*,5*S*)-2-methoxycarbonyltropan-3-yl benzoate; $C_{17}H_{21}NO_4$; relative molecular mass, 303

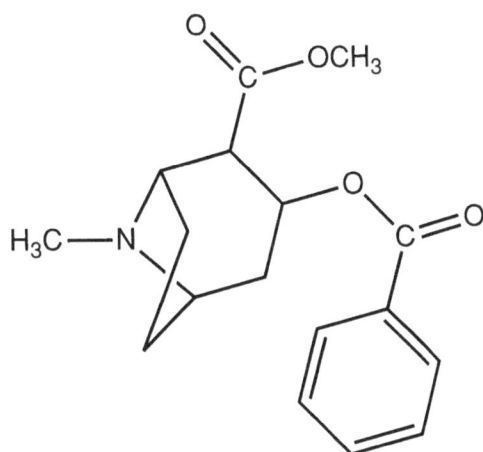

Cocaine is an alkaloid obtained from coca, the dried leaves of *Erythroxylon coca* and other species of *Erythroxylon*, or by synthesis from ecgonine. The hydrochloride salt is an effective local anaesthetic when used at concentrations of 10–200 g/l, but is normally only applied topically because of the risk of systemic toxicity if given by other routes.

Cocaine is frequently abused by injection or inhalation (sniffing, snorting) into the nasal passages; ingested cocaine has less effect owing to hydrolysis in the gastrointestinal tract. Cocaine free-base (crack) is very rapidly absorbed when inhaled into the nasal passages or smoked. The estimated minimum fatal dose in an adult is 1–2 g, but addicts may tolerate up to 5 g/day. The principal metabolites are benzoylecgonine, ecgonine and ecgonine methyl ester. Only 1–9% of an intravenous dose is excreted in urine as cocaine, while 35–55% is excreted as benzoylecgonine.

There is no simple qualitative test for cocaine, but this compound and its metabolites can be detected and identified by thin-layer chromatography of a basic solvent extract of urine (see section 5.2.3).

Clinical interpretation

Acute cocaine poisoning may cause euphoria, restlessness, vomiting, pyrexia, mydriasis, delirium, tremor, hyperreflexia, hypertension, hyperventilation, convulsions and cardiorespiratory failure. Treatment is symptomatic and supportive.

6.33 Codeine

Morphine methyl ether; 3-*O*-methylmorphine monohydrate; $C_{18}H_{21}NO_3 \cdot H_2O$; relative molecular mass, 317

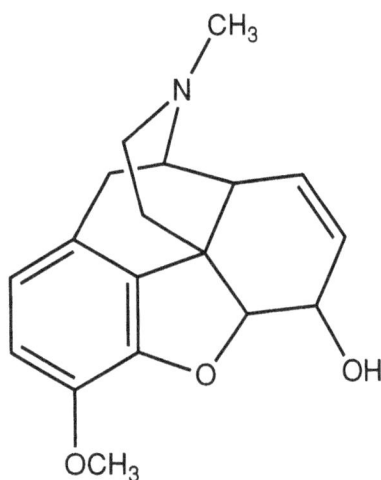

Codeine is a narcotic analgesic obtained either from opium or by methylation of morphine. Codeine is metabolized by *O*-demethylation and *N*-demethylation to give morphine and norcodeine, respectively, and by conjugation to form glucuronides and sulfates of both parent drug and metabolites. The estimated fatal dose of codeine in an adult is 800 mg. However, codeine is much less toxic than morphine, and death directly attributable to codeine is rare.

There is no simple qualitative test for codeine, but this compound and norcodeine can be detected and identified by thin-layer chromatography of a basic solvent extract of urine (see section 5.2.3).

Clinical interpretation

Acute overdosage with codeine gives rise to pinpoint pupils, hypotension, hypothermia, coma, convulsions, pulmonary oedema and cardiac arrhythmias. Death may ensue from profound respiratory depression. Naloxone rapidly reverses the central toxic effects of codeine (see section 2.2.2).

6.34 Copper

Copper salts such as copper(II) sulfate, chloride, and carbonate and cuprammonium salts such as cuprammonium carbonate ($Cu(NH_3)_2CO_3$) are used as insecticides and fungicides. As with iron salts, copper salts often impart a blue or green colour to stomach contents. Cuprammonium salts are much more toxic than copper salts owing to rapid absorption and the intrinsic toxicity of the cuprammonium ion. Acute poisoning may also follow inhalation of metallic copper fumes or powder.

Qualitative test

Applicable to stomach contents and scene residues.

Reagents

1. Dithiooxamide in methanol (10 g/l).
2. Concentrated ammonium hydroxide (relative density 0.88).

Method

1. Slowly place 0.1 ml of sample on a filter-paper to give a spot no greater than 1 cm in diameter, drying with a hairdrier if necessary.
2. Expose the spot to ammonia fumes from concentrated ammonium hydroxide **in a fume cupboard**, and add 0.1 ml of dithiooxamide solution to the spot.

Results

Copper salts give an olive-green stain. Chromium salts also give a green stain, which is normally visible before the dithiooxamide is added. A number of other metals give yellow-brown or red-brown colours with this reagent.

Sensitivity

Copper, 1 mg/l.

Confirmatory test

Applicable to stomach contents and scene residues.

Reagents

1. Aqueous zinc acetate solution (10 g/l).
2. Ammonium mercurithiocyanate reagent. Mix 8 g of mercuric chloride and 9 g of ammonium thiocyanate in 100 ml of purified water.
3. Aqueous hydrochloric acid (0.01 mol/l).

Method

1. Place 0.1 ml of sample in a well of a porcelain spotting tile and add 0.05 ml of dilute hydrochloric acid.
2. Mix 0.1 ml of ammonium mercurithiocyanate reagent with 0.1 ml of zinc acetate solution and add to the sample in the well.

Result

A violet precipitate of zinc mercurithiocyanate forms in the presence of copper salts.

Sensitivity

Copper, 50 mg/l.

Quantitative assay

Applicable to plasma or serum (1 ml).

Reagents

1. Oxalyl dihydrazide reagent. Mix 8 ml of saturated aqueous oxalyl dihydrazide, 12 ml of concentrated ammonium hydroxide (relative density 0.88), 20 ml of aqueous acetaldehyde (400 ml/l) and 20 ml of purified water.
2. Aqueous trichloroacetic acid (200 g/l).
3. Aqueous hydrochloric acid (2 mol/l).

Standards

Dissolve 1.00 g of copper foil, mesh or wire in a minimum volume of nitric acid (500 ml/l) and make up to 1 litre with dilute nitric acid (10 ml/l). Dilute portions of this solution with water to give solutions containing copper ion concentrations of 1.0, 2.0 and 5.0 mg/l.

Method

1. Add 0.7 ml of dilute hydrochloric acid to 1 ml of sample or standard in a plastic centrifuge tube, mix and allow to stand for 15 minutes.
2. Add 1 ml of trichloroacetic acid solution and mix thoroughly.
3. Allow to stand for 15 minutes and then centrifuge for 5 minutes.
4. Add 3 ml of oxalyl dihydrazide reagent to 1 ml of supernatant, mix and allow to stand for 20 minutes.

Results

Read the absorbance of the solution at 542 nm against an aqueous blank (see section 4.5.2) carried through the procedure. Plot the absorbance of the standard solutions against copper concentration, and calculate the copper concentration in the sample. The calibration graph is linear for copper concentrations of 1–25 mg/l.

Sensitivity

Copper, 1 mg/l.

Clinical interpretation

Ingestion of copper or cuprammonium salts leads initially to gastrointestinal symptoms (metallic taste, nausea, vomiting, epigastric pain and diarrhoea). In severe cases, hepatic damage (particularly in children), renal damage, haemolysis, coma and circulatory collapse may ensue. Normal serum copper concentrations are 0.7–1.6 mg/l, but in severe acute poisoning concentrations greater than 5 mg/l may be attained. Treatment is symptomatic and supportive, but may also include chelation therapy.

6.35 Coumarin anticoagulants

Phenprocoumon (4-hydroxy-3-(1-phenylpropyl)coumarin; $C_{18}H_{16}O_3$; relative molecular mass, 280) and warfarin (4-hydroxy-3-(3-oxo-1-phenylbutyl)coumarin; $C_{19}H_{16}O_4$; relative molecular mass, 308) are substituted 4-hydroxycoumarins.

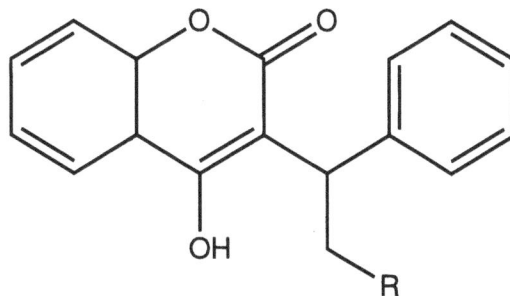

R = CH_3 (phenprocoumon)
R = $CO.CH_3$ (warfarin)

These compounds are widely used therapeutic agents; warfarin is also used as a rodenticide. Both inhibit blood coagulation by interfering with the synthesis of vitamin-K-dependent clotting factors. Their action is cumulative so that toxicity normally results from chronic administration. In contrast, severe toxicity may occur following a single large dose of a "superwarfarin" rodenticide such as difenacoum or brodifacoum.

115

The prothrombin time (see section 3.2.1) provides a simple, but nonspecific, means of measuring the severity of acute anticoagulant poisoning and of monitoring treatment. The simple method given below can be used to assess plasma phenprocoumon and warfarin concentrations.

Qualitative test
Applicable to plasma or serum (1.0 ml).

Reagents
1. Aqueous hydrochloric acid (1 mol/l).
2. *n*-Butyl acetate:chloroform:aqueous formic acid (850 ml/l) (60:40:10).
3. Triethylamine (50 g/l) in *n*-hexane.
4. Silica gel thin-layer chromatography plate (20 × 20 cm, 20 μm average particle size; see section 4.4.1).

Standards
Serum containing phenprocoumon or warfarin concentrations of 0, 1, 5 and 10 mg/l.

Method
1. To 1.0 ml of sample or standard add 0.9 ml of dilute hydrochloric acid, 0.1 ml of acetone and 5 ml of chloroform.
2. Mix for 2 minutes on a mechanical shaker and then centrifuge for 10 minutes.
3. Remove the upper (aqueous) layer, filter the extract through phase-separating filter-paper and evaporate to dryness under a stream of compressed air or nitrogen.

Thin-layer chromatography
1. Dissolve the residues in 50 μl of chloroform, spot on the plate, and develop (10-cm run) in *n*-butyl acetate:chloroform:formic acid (saturated tank; see section 4.4.3).
2. Allow the solvent to evaporate completely, develop again in triethylamine:*n*-hexane, and inspect under ultraviolet light (366 nm).

Results
Warfarin (hR_f about 87) shows a dark purple fluorescence, phenprocoumon (hR_f about 95) a brighter purple. The plasma concentrations of either compound can be assessed by comparison with the results obtained from the standards.

Sensitivity

Warfarin or phenprocoumon, 0.5 mg/l.

Clinical interpretation

Features of acute poisoning with anticoagulants include the occurrence of petechiae, spontaneous bruising, haematoma formation and frank haemorrhage, especially from the genitourinary and gastrointestinal tracts. Serum concentrations of either compound greater than 5 mg/l are often accompanied by haemorrhagic complications. Phenprocoumon and warfarin have long plasma half-lives (6–7 days and 0.5–3 days, respectively), and patients with high serum concentrations should be treated promptly. Therapy consists of vitamin K supplementation until a prothrombin time in the normal range is obtained. In very serious cases, intravenous administration of fresh frozen plasma or purified clotting factors may be considered.

6.36 Cyanide

Cyanide (CN^-) poisoning may be encountered after the inhalation of hydrogen cyanide (HCN) or after the ingestion of hydrocyanic acid or potassium or sodium cyanide. Complex cyanide solutions are used in metal electroplating and acidification of such solutions often leads to the release of hydrogen cyanide. Cyanogenic glycosides and other nitrile-containing compounds, such as amygdalin, which release cyanide *in vivo* occur in a number of plant tissues, including peach and apricot kernels, cassava root and lima beans.

Thiocyanate insecticides (ethyl thiocyanate, methyl thiocyanate) are also metabolized to cyanide ion *in vivo* and can cause serious toxicity. Cyanide is also a metabolite of sodium nitroprusside (used as a vasodilator) and some other nitrile-containing compounds, but cyanide poisoning is unusual in such cases. Inorganic thiocyanates and ferricyanide and ferrocyanide salts do not give rise to cyanide *in vivo* and are relatively nontoxic.

The qualitative test described below is based on the formation of a blue ferriferrocyanide complex (Prussian blue) with ferrous ions. Two microdiffusion methods (section 4.3.3) applicable to blood specimens are also given, both based on the liberation of hydrogen cyanide and subsequent formation of a coloured complex. The first, the *p*-nitro-benzaldehyde/*o*-dinitrobenzene method, can be used to give a rapid semiquantitative result, while the pyridine/barbituric acid method should be used for a full quantitative analysis.

Qualitative test

Applicable to stomach contents and scene residues. **Take care — specimens containing cyanides often evolve hydrogen cyanide if acidified**.

Reagents

1. Aqueous sodium hydroxide solution (100 g/l).
2. Aqueous ferrous sulfate solution (100 g/l, freshly prepared in freshly boiled and cooled water).
3. Aqueous hydrochloric acid (100 ml/l).

Method

1. Dilute 1 ml of sample with 2 ml of sodium hydroxide solution.
2. Add 2 ml of ferrous sulfate solution.
3. Add sufficient hydrochloric acid to dissolve the ferrous hydroxide precipitate.

Result

A blue colour indicates the presence of cyanide. There are no common sources of interference.

Sensitivity

Cyanide, 10 mg/l.

Quantitative assays

Applicable to heparinized whole blood (0.1–1.0 ml), which can be stored at 4 °C for 1–2 days if the analysis is delayed for any reason. (Cyanide in blood is less stable if stored at room temperature or at −20 °C.)

1. *p-Nitrobenzaldehyde/o-dinitrobenzene method*

Reagents

1. Aqueous sodium hydroxide (0.5 mol/l).
2. Aqueous sulfuric acid (3.6 mol/l).
3. *p*-Nitrobenzaldehyde (0.05 mol/l) in 2-methoxyethanol.
4. *o*-Dinitrobenzene (0.05 mol/l) in 2-methoxyethanol.

Standard

Aqueous potassium cyanide (10 mg/l, i.e., cyanide ion concentration, 4 mg/l).

Method

1. Take three microdiffusion cells (see section 4.3.3) and add to each of the centre wells:
   (a) 0.5 ml of *p*-nitrobenzaldehyde solution;
   (b) 0.5 ml of *o*-dinitrobenzene solution;
   (c) 0.1 ml of sodium hydroxide solution.
2. To the outer wells add 0.1 ml of:
   — purified water (cell 1);
   — potassium cyanide solution (cell 2);
   — test blood specimen (cell 3).
3. To each outer well add 0.5 ml of purified water and, on the opposite side of the outer well, 1.0 ml of dilute sulfuric acid.
4. Seal each well using silicone grease, and carefully mix the components of the outer wells.
5. Incubate at room temperature for 20 minutes and then add 1 ml of aqueous methanol (1:1) to the centre wells.
6. Transfer the contents of the centre wells to 5.0-ml volumetric flasks and make up to volume with aqueous methanol (1:1).

Results

The red coloration obtained with cyanide-containing solutions is stable for about 15 minutes. Measure the absorbance of the solutions from cells 2 and 3 at 560 nm against the purified water blank (cell 1; see section 4.5.2). Assess the cyanide ion concentration in the sample by comparison with the reading obtained from the standard.

Sensitivity

Cyanide, 0.5 mg/l.

2. *Pyridine/barbituric acid method*

Reagents

1. Aqueous sodium hydroxide (0.1 mol/l).
2. Aqueous chloramine T solution (2.5 g/l). (N.B. Solid chloramine T is not stable, and fresh supplies should be obtained frequently.)
3. Aqueous sodium hydrogen orthophosphate (1 mol/l).
4. Pyridine–barbituric acid reagent. Stir 6 g of barbituric acid (**not** diethyl barbituric acid, see section 6.9) into 6 ml of concentrated hydrochloric acid (relative density 1.18), and dilute with 30 ml of pyridine. Dilute the resulting solution to 100 ml with purified water. This solution must be freshly prepared.
5. Aqueous sulfuric acid (1 mol/l).

Standards

1. Cyanide stock solution. Dissolve 50 mg of potassium cyanide in 100 ml of aqueous sodium hydroxide (0.1 mol/l); cyanide ion concentration, 200 mg/l. **Take care when using concentrated cyanide solutions**.
2. Cyanide calibration solution. Dilute (1:99) the standard cyanide ion solution (200 mg/l) in aqueous sodium hydroxide (0.1 mol/l); final cyanide ion concentration 2 mg/l.

Method

1. Label seven microdiffusion cells (a) to (g) and add the reagents shown in Table 25 to the outer wells, reagent 5 (dilute sulfuric acid) being placed at the opposite side of the well to the others.
2. Add 2 ml of sodium hydroxide solution to each inner well, seal the cells with silicone grease, carefully mix the contents of the outer wells and incubate at room temperature for 4 hours.
3. Pipette 1.0 ml of the sodium hydroxide solution from each of the inner wells into prelabelled, stoppered test-tubes.
4. Add the following reagents sequentially and shake to mix:
   (a) 2 ml of phosphate buffer;
   (b) 1 ml of chloramine T solution;
   (c) 3 ml of pyridine–barbituric acid reagent.
5. Allow to stand for 10 minutes at room temperature.

Results

The presence of cyanide is indicated by a red/blue colour. Measure the absorbance at 587 nm of each solution against the purified water blank (section 4.5.2), diluting if necessary to bring the test reading on to the

Table 25. Cyanide measurement by microdiffusion: outer well reagent additions

Cell	Cyanide calibration solution (ml)	Water (ml)	Sulfuric acid (ml)	Blood (ml)
(a) Reagent blank	—	2.0	0.5	—
(b) Test specimen	—	1.0	0.5	1.0
(c) Test specimen	—	1.0	0.5	1.0
(d) Cyanide, 0.2 mg/l	0.1	1.9	0.5	—
(e) Cyanide, 1.0 mg/l	0.5	1.5	0.5	—
(f) Cyanide, 2.0 mg/l	1.0	1.0	0.5	—
(g) Cyanide, 4.0 mg/l	2.0	—	0.5	—

scale. Construct a calibration graph using the results obtained from the standard cyanide solutions and calculate the cyanide concentration in the sample.

Sensitivity
Cyanide, 0.2 mg/l.

Clinical interpretation

Acute cyanide poisoning is characterized by ataxia, headache, anxiety, dyspnoea, confusion, coma, collapse, metabolic acidosis, pulmonary oedema and respiratory arrest. Cyanosis may not be present. Supportive treatment includes the administration of oxygen. A number of antidotes have been used, including dicobalt edetate, hydroxocobalamin, sodium nitrite and sodium thiosulfate.

In serious poisoning with cyanide salts or hydrocyanic acid, blood cyanide ion concentrations are usually of the order of 2–10 mg/l. The qualitative test described above has insufficient sensitivity to detect these concentrations and should only be used for stomach contents and scene residues. Quantitative cyanide measurements have little immediate relevance to the treatment of acute poisoning since, to have any hope of success, therapy must be commenced as soon as possible.

Cyanide may also be present in the blood of fire victims owing to inhalation of hydrogen cyanide from the partial combustion of wool, silk and synthetic polymers such as polyurethanes and polyacrylonitriles. In such cases, blood cyanide concentrations may range from 0.2 to 1.0 mg/l. Carbon monoxide is usually also present. Blood cyanide concentrations in heavy cigarette smokers may be as high as 0.3 mg/l.

6.37 Dapsone

Bis(4-aminophenyl)sulfone; $C_{12}H_{12}N_2O_2S$; relative molecular mass, 248

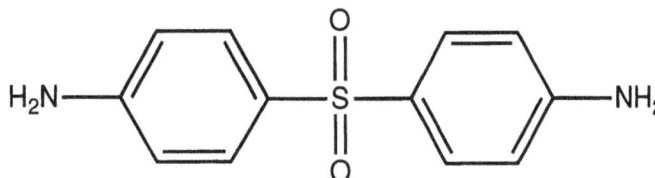

Dapsone is a structural analogue of the sulfonamide antibacterials and is used in the treatment of leprosy and dermatitis herpetiformis. Dapsone is metabolized to monoacetyldapsone, which also occurs in plasma, and to a variety of other products which are largely excreted in urine. Enterohepatic recirculation also occurs. In an adult, death may ensue 4–6 days after the ingestion of 1.5–5 g of dapsone.

The qualitative test described below can be used to give an estimate of the plasma dapsone concentration, if used with the appropriate standard solutions.

Qualitative test

Applicable to plasma or serum (0.5 ml).

Reagents

1. Aqueous sodium hydroxide (1 mol/l).
2. Chloroform:ethanol:glacial acetic acid (90:10:5).
3. Silica gel thin-layer chromatography plate (10 × 20 cm, 20 µm average particle size, see section 4.4.1).

Standards

Solutions containing dapsone concentrations of 5, 10, 20 and 50 mg/l in blank plasma, prepared by dilution from a methanolic stock solution (dapsone 1.00 g/l).

Method

1. Add 0.5 ml of sample or standard to 0.2 ml of sodium hydroxide solution and 6 ml of chloroform in a test-tube with a ground-glass stopper.
2. Stopper the tube, vortex-mix for 30 seconds and centrifuge for 5 minutes.
3. Discard the upper, aqueous layer, transfer 5 ml of the chloroform extract to a second tube and evaporate to dryness under a stream of compressed air or nitrogen.

Thin-layer chromatography

1. Reconstitute the extracts in 50 µl of methanol and spot on the plate. Spot extracts of the standard dapsone solutions on adjacent columns on the plate.
2. Develop the chromatogram (10-cm run) with chloroform: ethanol:glacial acetic acid (saturated tank, section 4.4.3).
3. Remove the plate, allow to dry and inspect under ultraviolet light (254 nm).

Results

Estimate the dapsone concentration in the sample by comparison with the results from the standard solutions. hR_f values: dapsone, 57; mono-acetyldapsone, 40.

Sensitivity

Dapsone, 2 mg/l.

Clinical interpretation

Ingestion of dapsone may cause anorexia, nausea, vomiting, abdominal pain, headache, tinnitus and blurred vision, with dizziness, agitation, coma and convulsions in severe cases. Haemolytic anaemia, methaemoglobinaemia, haematuria, jaundice and acute renal failure are further complications.

Plasma dapsone concentrations of 10 mg/l or more may be associated with toxicity. Repeat-dose oral activated charcoal is probably the most effective method of treatment, but methylene blue and exchange transfusion may be needed to treat methaemoglobinaemia and haemolytic anaemia, respectively.

6.38 Dextropropoxyphene

(+)-Propoxyphene; (+)-(1S,2R)-1-benzyl-3-dimethylamino-2-methyl-1-phenylpropyl propionate; $C_{22}H_{29}NO_2$; relative molecular mass, 340

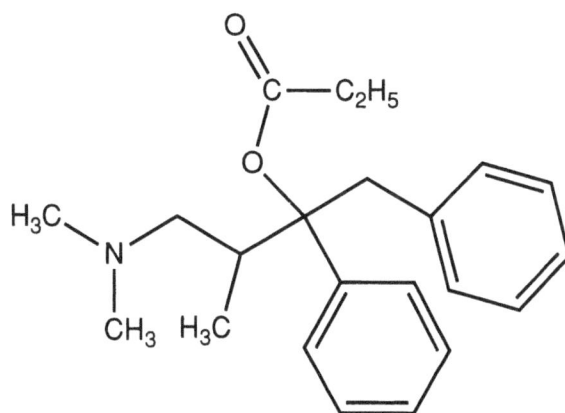

Dextropropoxyphene is a narcotic analgesic structurally related to methadone, and is often formulated together with paracetamol. Dextropropoxyphene is extensively metabolized to *N*-desmethyldextropropoxyphene (nordextropropoxyphene), which is the principal urinary metabolite.

There is no simple qualitative test for dextropropoxyphene, but this compound and its metabolites can be detected and identified by thin-layer chromatography of a basic solvent extract of urine (see section 5.2.3). In addition, paracetamol can be detected in urine using the *o*-cresol/ammonia test (see section 6.83).

Clinical interpretation

Acute overdosage with dextropropoxyphene gives rise to pin-point pupils, hypotension, hypothermia, coma, pulmonary oedema, convulsions and cardiac arrhythmias. Death may ensue rapidly from profound respiratory depression, especially if ethanol is also present. Naloxone rapidly reverses the central toxic effects of dextropropoxyphene (see section 2.2.2).

6.39 Dichloralphenazone

A stoichiometric complex of chloral hydrate and phenazone, $C_{15}H_{18}Cl_6N_2O_5$; relative molecular mass, 519

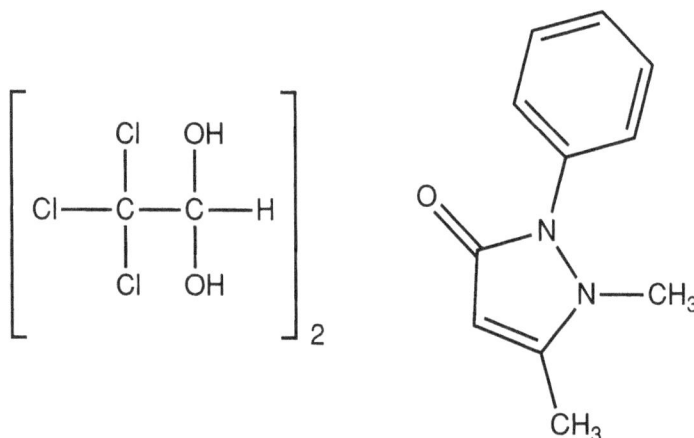

Dichloralphenazone is a mild hypnotic and acts as a mixture of each of its components, chloral hydrate and phenazone, *in vivo*. Dichloralphenazone ingestion can therefore be detected in urine using the Fujiwara test for the chloral metabolite trichloroacetic acid. Phenazone does not possess hypnotic activity and can be detected by thin-layer chromatography of a basic/neutral extract of urine (see section 5.2.3), using acidified iodoplatinate reagent only.

Qualitative test

Applicable to urine. Fujiwara test — see carbon tetrachloride monograph (section 6.23).

Results

An intense red/purple colour in the upper, pyridine layer indicates the presence of trichloro compounds. The blank analysis excludes contamination with chloroform from the laboratory atmosphere.

This test is very sensitive and will detect ingestion of a therapeutic dose of dichloralphenazone or chloral hydrate 12–24 hours later. However, other compounds, notably the solvent trichloroethylene, also give rise to trichloroacetic acid *in vivo*, so that caution must be exercised in reporting results.

Sensitivity
Trichloroacetate, 1 mg/l.

Clinical interpretation

Acute poisoning with dichloralphenazone can cause vomiting, excitement, ataxia, confusion, drowsiness, stupor, hypotension, coma, cardiac arrhythmias, respiratory depression and pulmonary oedema. Treatment is normally symptomatic and supportive.

6.40 Dichloromethane

Methylene chloride; CH_2Cl_2; relative molecular mass, 85

Dichloromethane is widely used in paint strippers, sometimes together with toluene, and as a laboratory and industrial solvent. Its acute toxicity is largely due to direct depressant effects on the central nervous system. Dichloromethane is partially metabolized to carbon monoxide, which may contribute to chronic toxicity.

There is no simple test for dichloromethane in biological samples. However, measurement of carboxyhaemoglobin saturation is important in the assessment of chronic exposure to dichloromethane. Urine samples from patients exposed to dichloromethane do not give a positive result with the Fujiwara test.

Clinical interpretation

Exposure to dichloromethane may cause dizziness, numbness, irritability, fatigue, nausea, hypoventilation, pulmonary oedema and respiratory arrest. Recovery is normally rapid once the patient is removed from the contaminated atmosphere. Supplemental oxygen may be indicated, especially if features of carbon monoxide poisoning are present.

6.41 Digoxin and digitoxin

Digoxin ($C_{41}H_{64}O_{14}$; relative molecular mass, 781) and digitoxin ($C_{41}H_{64}O_{13}$; relative molecular mass, 765) are cardioactive glycosides obtained from the leaves of certain species of *Digitalis* (e.g. foxglove). Digoxin is widely used as an antiarrhythmic. Cardiac glycosides are also used as euthanasia agents in veterinary practice in certain countries. These compounds are very potent and there is no simple method for detecting them in blood or urine.

Qualitative test

Applicable to stomach contents and scene residues.

Reagents

1. Silica gel thin-layer chromatography plate (10 × 20 cm, 20 μm average particle size; see section 4.4.1).
2. Toluene:ethanol (7:3).
3. Chloramine T reagent. Mix 10 ml of aqueous chloramine T (30 g/l) and 40 ml of methanol containing 250 g/l trichloroacetic acid.
4. Aqueous perchloric acid (150 g/l).

Standards

Digoxin and digitoxin (both 100 mg/l) in chloroform.

Method

1. Add 5 ml of chloroform to 1 ml of sample, vortex-mix for 30 seconds and centrifuge for 5 minutes.
2. Discard the upper, aqueous layer and filter the chloroform extract through phase-separating filter-paper into a clean tube.
3. Evaporate the extract to dryness under a stream of compressed air or nitrogen and reconstitute in 50 μl of chloroform.

Thin-layer chromatography

1. Divide the plate into two halves and spot 20 μl of the reconstituted extract and 10 μl of the standard solutions on to columns on both halves of the plate.
2. Develop the chromatogram (10-cm run) using toluene:ethanol (saturated tank, see section 4.4.3).
3. Allow the plate to dry, and spray one half of the plate with chloramine T reagent and the other half with perchloric acid solution.
4. Heat the plate in an oven at 100 °C for 10 minutes.

Results

hR_f values and colour reactions with the spray reagents are listed in Table 26.

Sensitivity

Digoxin or digitoxin, 10 mg/l.

Clinical interpretation

Digoxin and digitoxin are potent cardiotoxins and can give rise to fatal arrhythmias. Nausea, vomiting, diarrhoea, drowsiness and confusion

Table 26. Thin-layer chromatography of digoxin and digitoxin: hR$_f$ values and colour reactions

Compound	hR$_f$	Chloramine T reagent		Perchloric acid (150 g/l)	
		Visible	Ultraviolet (366 nm)	Visible	Ultraviolet (366 nm)
Digoxin	62	Brown ring	Blue-green	Grey	Blue-green
Digitoxin	72	—	—	Brown	Dark brown

occur in the early stages of poisoning with these compounds. Hyperkalaemia and tachyarrhythmias are characteristic of severe poisoning. Treatment is generally supportive. Antigen-binding (F$_{ab}$) antibody fragments will reverse toxicity in digoxin poisoning (see section 2.2.2), but are indicated only in very severe cases.

6.42 Dinitrophenol pesticides

These compounds have the general structure:

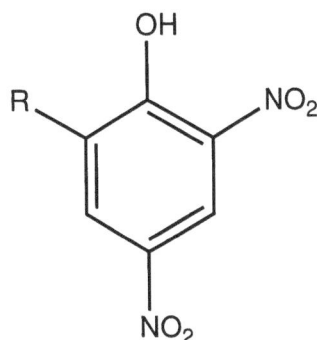

The dinitrophenols most commonly encountered are DNOC (2-methyl-4,6-dinitrophenol; 4,6,-dinitro-o-cresol; C$_7$H$_6$N$_2$O$_5$; relative molecular mass, 198) and dinoseb (2-sec-butyl-4,6-dinitrophenol; C$_{10}$H$_{12}$N$_2$O$_5$; relative molecular mass, 240). DNOC is used as an insecticide and as a herbicide on fruit trees, while dinoseb is used mostly as a herbicide. Severe dinitrophenol poisoning may follow occupational exposure as well as ingestion. Skin is a common route of absorption and intense yellow staining may be diagnostic.

Both DNOC and dinoseb can be measured easily in whole blood since they show strong absorbance at 430 nm and the concentrations associated with toxicity are relatively high.

Quantitative assay

Applicable to whole blood (1 ml).

Reagents

1. Concentrated hydrochloric acid (relative density 1.18).
2. Aqueous sodium chloride (270 g/l) containing sodium carbonate (30 g/l).

Standards

Solutions containing dinitrophenol concentrations of 10, 20 and 50 mg/l in whole blood.

Method

1. Add 5 ml of butanone (methyl ethyl ketone) to 1 ml of sample or standard in a conical tube, and add 1 ml of the sodium chloride/ sodium carbonate solution.
2. Vortex-mix for 30 seconds, centrifuge for 5 minutes and transfer 2-ml portions of the extract to two clean tubes.
3. Add 50 μl of hydrochloric acid to one tube, vortex-mix for 10 seconds and centrifuge for 5 minutes.
4. Measure the difference in absorbance between the solutions at 430 nm (1-cm path-length cells).

Results

Construct a graph of the difference in absorbance against dinitrophenol concentration in the calibration solutions and calculate the dinitrophenol concentration in the sample.

Sensitivity

Dinitrophenol, 10 mg/l

Clinical interpretation

Dinitrophenols uncouple oxidative phosphorylation, and fatigue, excessive sweating, hyperthermia and thirst may be followed by exhaustion and death in severe cases. Toxic effects often appear at blood concentrations greater than 30 mg/l while concentrations greater than 60 mg/l are associated with severe toxicity.

6.43 Diphenhydramine

2-Benzhydryloxy-*N,N*-dimethylethylamine; $C_{17}H_{21}NO$; relative molecular mass, 255

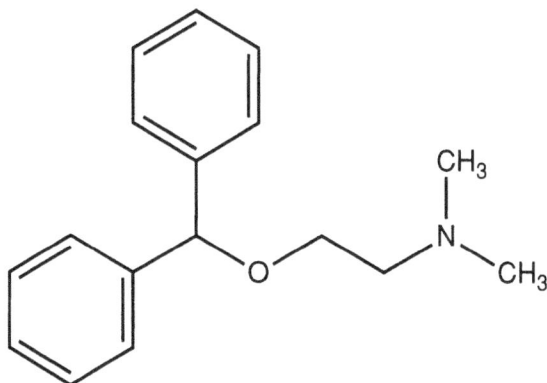

Diphenhydramine is a widely used antihistamine. Less than 1% of the dose is excreted unchanged but *N*-dealkylation, oxidative deamination and conjugation give rise to a number of compounds which are excreted in urine.

There is no simple qualitative test for diphenhydramine and its metabolites, but this compound can be detected and identified by thin-layer chromatography of a basic solvent extract of urine, stomach contents or scene residues (see section 5.2.3).

Clinical interpretation

Overdosage with diphenhydramine and other antihistamines may cause drowsiness, dizziness, dry mouth, headache, nausea, tachycardia, fever, hallucinations and tremor. In more severe cases, this may be followed by coma, convulsions and death. Treatment is symptomatic and supportive.

6.44 Diquat

1,1'-Ethylene-2,2'-bipyridylium ion; $C_{12}H_{12}N_2$; relative molecular mass, 184

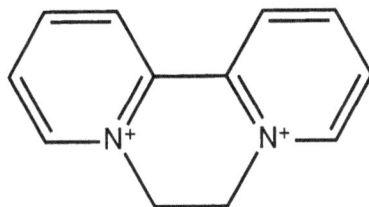

Diquat is a contact herbicide structurally related to paraquat, with which it is often formulated. Diquat is often encountered as the dibromide salt and death has been reported following the ingestion of as little as 2 g of diquat. Diquat and paraquat give highly coloured products with sodium dithionite, and this reaction forms the basis of the test described.

Qualitative test

Applicable to urine, stomach contents and scene residues.

Reagents

1. Sodium dithionite (solid, stored in a desiccator).
2. Aqueous ammonium hydroxide (2 mol/l).
3. Blank urine.
4. Urine specimen containing diquat ion (10 mg/l).

Method

1. Add 0.5 ml of ammonium hydroxide solution to the test solution and to the blank and standard urines (1-ml volumes) in separate test-tubes.
2. Add about 20 mg of sodium dithionite to each tube and mix.
3. If a colour forms in the test solution, agitate in air for several minutes.

Results

A yellow-green colour indicates diquat. Paraquat gives a blue/blue-black colour. This test cannot detect diquat in the presence of paraquat.

If the colour fades on continued agitation in air, diquat/paraquat is confirmed — the original colour can be restored by adding more sodium dithionite.

Sensitivity

Diquat, 5 mg/l.

Clinical interpretation

Ingestion of diquat may cause irritation of the mouth and throat, epigastric pain, vomiting, diarrhoea, intestinal paralysis, malaise, excitement, convulsions, coma and hepatorenal failure. Unlike paraquat, diquat does not cause progressive pulmonary fibrosis. Treatment is largely symptomatic and supportive.

6.45 Ephedrine

(1R,2S)-2-Methylamino-1-phenylpropan-1-ol hemihydrate; $C_{10}H_{15}NO \cdot (H_2O)_{1/2}$; relative molecular mass, 174

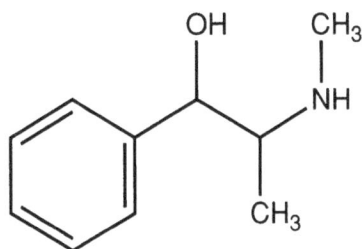

Ephedrine is a sympathomimetic agent. It is metabolized by *N*-demethylation to norephedrine (phenylpropanolamine), and by oxidative deamination and conjugation. Ephedrine is itself a metabolite of methylephedrine. The estimated minimum lethal dose of ephedrine in an adult is 4 g, but fatalities are rare.

There is no simple qualitative test for ephedrine, but this compound and its metabolites can be detected and identified by thin-layer chromatography of a basic solvent extract of urine (see section 5.2.3).

Clinical interpretation

Ephedrine overdosage may cause nausea, vomiting, headache, thirst, irritability, fever, tachycardia, sweating, dilated pupils, convulsions, coma and respiratory depression. Treatment is symptomatic and supportive.

6.46 Ethanol

Ethyl alcohol; alcohol; C_2H_5OH; relative molecular mass, 46

Acute poisoning with ethanol is very frequently encountered in hospital admissions and is usually the result of ingestion of alcoholic drinks. Poisoning with industrial alcohol (methylated spirit) containing various denaturants, notably methanol, also occurs.

The qualitative test described below will detect volatile reducing agents, of which ethanol is the most common. The quantitative assay is based on the oxidation of ethanol to acetaldehyde by alcohol dehydrogenase (ADH) in the presence of nicotinamide adenine dinucleotide (NAD), and is applicable to whole blood; if plasma or serum is used, the protein precipitation step with perchloric acid can be omitted. A number of manufacturers supply ethanol assay kits based on this reaction; if available, such kits often prove more economical than separate purchase of the reagents.

Qualitative test

Applicable to urine, stomach contents and scene residues.

Reagent

Potassium dichromate (25 g/l) in aqueous sulfuric acid (500 ml/l).

Method

1. Apply 50 μl of potassium dichromate solution to a strip of glass-fibre filter-paper and insert the paper in the neck of a test-tube containing 1 ml of sample.
2. Lightly stopper the tube and place in a boiling water-bath for 2 minutes.

Results

A change in colour from orange to green indicates the presence of volatile reducing agents such as ethanol (see plate 7); metaldehyde, methanol and paraldehyde also react.

Sensitivity

Ethanol, 0.5 g/l.

Quantitative assay

Applicable to whole blood, plasma, or serum (0.5 ml).

Reagents

1. Semicarbazide reagent. Dissolve 10 g of tetrasodium pyrophosphate decahydrate, 2.5 g of semicarbazide hydrochloride and 0.5 g of glycine in 250 ml of purified water. Add 10 ml of aqueous sodium hydroxide (2 mol/l) and dilute to 300 ml.
2. Aqueous nicotinamide adenine dinucleotide (NAD; also known as diphosphopyridine nucleotide, DPN) (13 g/l). This solution is stable for 2–3 months at 4 °C, but can be decomposed by vigorous agitation.
3. Alcohol dehydrogenase (ADH) suspension. Mix 45.5 g of ammonium sulfate and 3 g of tetrasodium pyrophosphate decahydrate in 100 ml of purified water adjusted to pH 7.3 (using a pH meter) with either aqueous hydrochloric acid or sodium hydroxide (both 1 mol/l) and containing 2.5 g of suspended crystalline yeast ADH; this solution is stable for 2–3 months at 4 °C.

4. Aqueous perchloric acid (2.9 ml of perchloric acid (700 ml/l) in 100 ml of purified water).

Standards

Solutions containing ethanol concentrations of 0.5, 1.0, 2.0 and 4.0 g/l prepared in heparinized whole blood to which 10 g/l sodium fluoride has been added. These solutions are stable for up to 1 month if stored at 4 °C in well-sealed containers.

Method

1. Add 0.5 ml of blood to 2 ml of perchloric acid solution in a test-tube.
2. Vortex-mix for 30 seconds and then centrifuge for 5 minutes.
3. Add 0.1 ml of the supernatant (or 0.2 ml of an aqueous dilution (1:9) of plasma/serum) to a 10-ml tube containing 4.5 ml of semicarbazide reagent and vortex-mix for 10 seconds.
4. Add 0.1 ml of NAD solution and 0.02 ml of ADH suspension and mix gently so as not to cause foaming.
5. Allow to stand for 70 minutes at 20–25 °C and measure the absorbance at 340 nm against a reagent blank (see section 4.5.3).

Results

Construct a calibration graph of absorbance against blood ethanol concentration by analysis of the standard ethanol solutions and calculate the concentration of ethanol in the sample.

If the specimen contains an ethanol concentration of more than 4.0 g/l, the analysis should be repeated using a dilution (1:1 or 1:3) of the sample in blank plasma. Methanol does not interfere, but propan-2-ol and some higher alcohols will reduce NAD under the conditions used in this assay.

In all cases where the analysis may be delayed, it is important to add 10 g/l sodium fluoride to the specimen to inhibit microbial metabolism (see section 5.1.6).

Sensitivity

Ethanol, 0.5 g/l.

Clinical interpretation

Ethanol is rapidly absorbed from the small intestine and can cause disinhibition, blurred vision, drowsiness, incoordination and confusion, with nausea, vomiting and coma in severe cases. Hypoglycaemia and convulsions may also occur, especially in young children. Treatment of acute poisoning is normally symptomatic and supportive, although dialysis may be considered in severe cases (see section 2.2.3).

A simple guide to the interpretation of blood ethanol results is given in Table 27. However, remember that (1) ethanol potentiates the depressant effects on the central nervous system of many other drugs, and (2) chronic alcoholics may show few features of intoxication even with blood ethanol concentrations of 4 g/l or more. Blood ethanol measurements are therefore rarely helpful in the management of acute poisoning with this compound.

Ethanol can be given to treat poisoning with ethylene glycol and methanol (see section 2.2.2), since it inhibits the production of toxic metabolites. Monitoring of the plasma ethanol concentrations attained is often useful in such cases, as noted in the appropriate monographs (sections 6.48 and 6.70).

Table 27. Interpretation of blood ethanol concentrations

Blood ethanol (g/l)	Clinical features (in non-habitual users of alcohol)
0.5	Flushed face, euphoria; usually little apparent clinical effect in adults. May be associated with hypoglycaemia in young children
1.0	Incoordination, speech defects
1.5	Marked incoordination, staggering gait, dilated pupils, nystagmus
3.0	Gross incoordination, stupor, vomiting
5.0	Coma

6.47 Ethchlorvynol

1-Chloro-3-ethylpent-1-en-4-yn-3-ol; C_7H_9ClO; relative molecular mass, 145

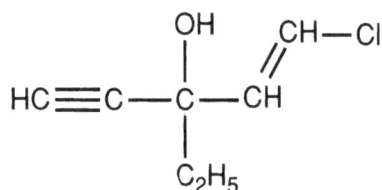

Ethchlorvynol is a nonbarbiturate hypnotic with a pungent smell. The test described is based on the reaction between ethchlorvynol and diphenylamine in the presence of concentrated sulfuric acid.

Qualitative test

Applicable to urine, stomach contents and scene residues.

Reagents

1. Diphenylamine sulfate (solid).
2. Concentrated sulfuric acid (relative density 1.83).

Method

1. Add about 20 mg of diphenylamine sulfate crystals to the surface of 2 ml of test solution in a glass test-tube.
2. **Slowly** add 1 ml of sulfuric acid down the side of the tube.

Results

A bright red colour on the surface of the crystals indicates the presence of ethchlorvynol. This test is specific and will detect a therapeutic dosage of ethchlorvynol if performed on urine.

Sensitivity

Ethchlorvynol, 1 mg/l.

Clinical interpretation

Ingestion of ethchlorvynol may cause fatigue, headache, confusion, nausea, vomiting, coma and respiratory depression. Treatment is symptomatic and supportive.

6.48 Ethylene glycol

Ethane-1,2-diol; glycol; $CH_2OH.CH_2OH$; relative molecular mass, 62

Ethylene glycol is used mainly in vehicle radiator antifreeze as a concentrated 200–500 ml/l aqueous solution, sometimes together with methanol. Ethylene glycol is itself relatively nontoxic, but is metabolized by alcohol dehydrogenase giving rise to glycolic and oxalic acids. Some of the later features observed in ethylene glycol poisoning are therefore characteristic of poisoning with oxalates. The potentially fatal dose of antifreeze containing ethylene glycol in an adult is 50–100 ml.

There is no simple method for the detection and identification of ethylene glycol in biological specimens. However, a rise in plasma osmolality is a useful but nonspecific indicator of poisoning with this compound (see section 3.1.3). Oxalic acid may be excreted in urine as calcium oxalate, and the tests for oxalates will detect this compound (see section 6.82). The crystalluria produced may also be diagnostic (see section 5.2.1).

Clinical interpretation

Ingestion of ethylene glycol may give rise initially to clinical features similar to those of ethanol intoxication, and inebriation, drowsiness, nausea, and vomiting may occur. Production of glycolate may give rise to a marked metabolic acidosis, which may help to indicate the diagnosis (see section 3.1.2). Oxalic acid itself sequesters calcium and hypocalcaemia, muscular twitching and tetany, convulsions, flank pain, acute renal failure and cardiac arrest are later features of severe ethylene glycol poisoning.

Plasma concentrations of ethylene glycol of 0.5 g/l or more are normally associated with serious poisoning, although the time of ingestion is important in interpreting results. Ethanol prevents metabolism of ethylene glycol by competitive inhibition of alcohol dehydrogenase. Treatment of ethylene glycol poisoning consists of correction of any metabolic acidosis and of hypocalcaemia, ethanol administration and peritoneal dialysis or haemodialysis to treat renal failure and remove unchanged ethylene glycol. Plasma ethanol concentrations of about 1 g/l should be attained and monitored to ensure they are maintained during treatment since dialysis removes this compound as well as ethylene glycol.

6.49 Fluoride

Hydrogen fluoride (hydrofluoric acid, HF) and inorganic fluoride salts are widely used in industry and in the fluoridation of water supplies. Sodium fluoride (NaF), sodium fluorosilicate (Na_2SiF_6), and cryolite (Na_3AlF_6) are employed as insecticides and rodenticides. Fluorides are also used as preservatives, and in dentifrices and toothpastes. The estimated lethal dose of sodium fluoride in an adult is 1–4 g. Young children may ingest up to 0.5 g of fluoride by swallowing fluoride toothpaste.

The simple tests for fluorine-containing compounds given below will also detect fluoroacetates such as fluoroacetamide and sodium fluoroacetate. Fluoride ion can be measured reliably in blood and urine by use of a fluoride-selective electrode. Alternatively, the microdiffusion technique (see section 4.3.3) described below can be used. This relies on the liberation of HF from the sample; polypropylene vessels must be used, since HF attacks glass.

Qualitative test
Applicable to urine, stomach contents and scene residues.

Reagents

1. Aqueous sodium chloride solution (50 g/l).
2. Concentrated sulfuric acid (relative density 1.83).
3. Solid calcium hydroxide.
4. Powdered silica (silicon dioxide, SiO_2).

Method

1. Place 5 ml of sample in a porcelain crucible (10-ml volume), add 100 mg of calcium hydroxide and evaporate gently to dryness over a microburner.
2. To destroy organic material, heat strongly until a white ash remains.
3. Add 200 mg of powdered silica and mix with the residue, stirring and scraping the sides of the crucible.
4. Spot 100 μl of sodium chloride solution on to a glass microscope slide. Add 1 ml of concentrated sulfuric acid to the crucible and quickly cover with the slide, inverted so that the sodium chloride solution is suspended over the crucible.
5. Place a small beaker containing ice on the slide and heat the crucible gently over the microburner for 5 minutes.
6. Remove the slide and examine the sodium chloride solution under a low-power microscope.

Results

Volatile silicon tetrafluoride dissolves in the suspended drop to form sodium silicon tetrafluoride. As the water evaporates from the slide this forms small hexagonal crystals, sometimes with a pinkish tinge, which appear at the edge of the drop and before any larger, cubic sodium chloride crystals. This is a general test for fluorine-containing compounds, but is relatively insensitive.

Sensitivity

Fluoride, 100 mg/l.

Confirmatory test

Applicable to urine, stomach contents and scene residues.

Reagents

1. Concentrated sulfuric acid (relative density 1.83).
2. Solid calcium hydroxide.
3. Paraffin wax.

Method

1. Place 5 ml of sample in a 10-ml porcelain crucible, add 100 mg of calcium hydroxide and evaporate gently to dryness over a micro-burner.
2. To destroy organic material, heat strongly until a white ash remains.
3. Smear paraffin wax on to a glass microscope slide and scratch out a symbol (X) to expose part of the glass.
4. Add 1 ml of concentrated sulfuric acid to the crucible and quickly cover with the slide, inverted so that the exposed glass is over the crucible.
5. Remove the slide after 20 minutes and clean off the remaining wax with a solvent such as toluene.

Results

If fluorinated compounds are present, hydrogen fluoride is generated, which etches the exposed glass. This is a general test for fluorine-containing compounds, but is relatively insensitive.

Sensitivity

Fluoride, 100 mg/l.

Quantitative assay

Applicable to whole blood, plasma or serum.

Reagents

1. Aqueous sulfuric acid (800 ml/l) containing 2.5 g/l tergitol.
2. Aqueous cerous nitrate solution (432 mg/l).
3. Alizarin reagent. Mix 38.5 mg of alizarin complexone, 4.2 ml of glacial acetic acid and 2.2 g of anhydrous sodium acetate with 100 ml of purified water, final pH 4.3.
4. Polypropylene microdiffusion vessels, Öbrink's modification, which has a sealing well, in addition to the inner and outer wells (size 68).[a]

Standards

Aqueous solutions of sodium fluoride containing fluoride ion concentrations of 0.5, 1.0 and 5.0 mg/l.

---

[a]Conway polypropylene diffusion cells, Bel-Art Products, Pequannock, NJ 07440, USA.

Method

1. To each microdiffusion cell add:

   (a) 1.5 ml of sulfuric acid solution to the sealing well;
   (b) 1.0 ml of sample or standard and 1.0 ml of sulfuric acid solution, **without mixing**, to the outer well;
   (c) 0.25 ml of cerous nitrate solution and 0.25 ml of alizarin reagent to the centre well.

2. Seal the cells, gently mix the contents of the outer wells and allow to stand for 3 hours at room temperature.

Results

A blue colour in the centre well indicates the presence of fluoride. The fluoride concentration in the sample can be estimated by comparison with the results obtained on analysis of the standard fluoride solutions.

Sensitivity

Fluoride, 0.5 mg/l.

Clinical interpretation

Inhalation of hydrogen fluoride may cause coughing, choking, fever, dyspnoea, cyanosis and pulmonary oedema. Ingestion of hydrofluoric acid may cause nausea, vomiting, diarrhoea and abdominal pain, while skin contact may give deep and painful ulceration. Systemic toxic effects include weakness, tetany, convulsions, respiratory depression and acute hepatorenal failure. Treatment is symptomatic and may include intensive supportive measures.

Ingestion of fluoride salts may give rise to a burning sensation in the mouth and throat, dysphagia, thirst, excessive salivation, vomiting and diarrhoea. In severe cases muscle cramps, weakness and tremor may be followed by respiratory and cardiac failure. Plasma fluoride concentrations are normally less than 0.2 mg/l; urine concentrations are usually less than 1 mg/l, but up to 4 mg/l is not considered harmful. Blood concentrations of 2.6 mg/l or more have been recorded in fatalities.

6.50 Fluoroacetate

Sodium fluoroacetate ($CF_3.COONa$) and fluoroacetamide ($CF_3.CONH_2$) are used mainly as rodenticides. Fluoroacetic acid is the toxic principle of *Dichapetalum cymosum* (gifblaar), a plant endemic to southern Africa. Fluoroacetates block the tricarboxylic acid cycle and are extremely toxic — the approximate lethal oral dose for adults is 30 mg.

Both the qualitative tests described below rely on the generation and subsequent detection of volatile fluorine derivatives from fluoroacetates present in the sample.

Qualitative test

Applicable to stomach contents and scene residues. See fluoride monograph (section 6.49).

Results

Volatile silicon tetrafluoride dissolves in the suspended drop to form sodium silicon tetrafluoride. As the water evaporates from the slide this forms small hexagonal crystals, sometimes with a pinkish tinge, which appear at the edge of the drop and before any larger, cubic sodium chloride crystals. This is a general test for fluorine-containing compounds, but is relatively insensitive.

Sensitivity

Fluoroacetate, 100 mg/l.

Confirmatory test

Applicable to stomach contents and scene residues.
See fluoride monograph (section 6.49).

Results

If fluorinated compounds are present, hydrogen fluoride is generated, which etches the exposed glass. This is a general test for fluorine-containing compounds, but is relatively insensitive.

Sensitivity

Fluoroacetate, 100 mg/l.

Clinical interpretation

Exposure to fluoroacetates may cause nausea and apprehension, which may be followed by tremor, cardiac arryhthmias, convulsions and coma. The onset of symptoms may be delayed by 0.5–2 hours. Death occurs from respiratory and cardiac failure, often associated with pulmonary oedema. Treatment is symptomatic and supportive.

6.51 Formaldehyde

Formaldehyde (HCHO; relative molecular mass, 30) is a colourless, inflammable gas and is normally encountered as an aqueous solution (formalin, 340–380 ml/l), which also contains methanol as a stabilizer. Formalin is used as a disinfectant, an antiseptic and a tissue-fixing and embalming fluid. Polymerized formaldehyde (paraformaldehyde) is used as a fumigant, and other polymeric forms are used as adhesives in chipboard and plywood, and in the preparation of insulation materials.

Formaldehyde is rapidly metabolized *in vivo* to formate and is itself a metabolite of methanol. Acute formaldehyde poisoning is uncommon, but 30 ml of formalin may be fatal in an adult.

Qualitative test
Applicable to stomach contents and scene residues.

Reagents
1. Concentrated sulfuric acid (relative density 1.83).
2. Chromotropic acid (solid).

Method
1. Add about 100 mg of chromotropic acid to 0.5 ml of test solution and vortex-mix for 5 seconds.
2. **Carefully** add 1.5 ml of concentrated sulfuric acid.

Results
A purple-violet colour indicates the presence of formaldehyde.

Sensitivity
Formaldehyde, 20 mg/l.

Clinical interpretation
Formaldehyde vapour is very irritating and inhalation may cause conjunctivitis, coughing and laryngeal and pulmonary oedema. Ingestion of formaldehyde solution may give rise to abdominal pain, vomiting, diarrhoea, hypotension, coma, metabolic acidosis and acute renal failure. Treatment is normally symptomatic and supportive.

6.52 Formic acid and formate

Formic acid (HCOOH; relative molecular mass, 46), a colourless, aqueous solution, is very corrosive. Many proprietary descaling agents contain 500–600 ml/l formic acid. Formates such as sodium formate (HCOONa) are used as synthetic intermediates and in the dying, printing and tanning industries. Formic acid is itself a metabolite of methanol and formaldehyde. The minimum lethal dose of formic acid in an adult is thought to be about 30 ml.

The initial test given below should be used if formic acid is suspected. In the confirmatory test both formic acid and formates are reduced to formaldehyde, which can then be detected by reaction with chromotropic acid.

Qualitative test

Applicable to stomach contents and scene residues.

Reagents

1. Citric acid/acetamide reagent. Citric acid (5 g/l) and acetamide (100 g/l) in propan-2-ol.
2. Aqueous sodium acetate (300 g/l).
3. Acetic anhydride.

Method

1. Add 0.5 ml of test solution to 1 ml of citric acid/acetamide reagent and then add 0.1 ml of sodium acetate solution and 3.5 ml of acetic anhydride.
2. Vortex-mix for 5 seconds and heat in a boiling water-bath for 10 minutes.

Results

A red colour indicates the presence of formic acid. Formaldehyde and formate salts do not react in this test.

Sensitivity

Formic acid, 50 mg/l.

Confirmatory test

Applicable to stomach contents and scene residues.

Reagents

1. Aqueous hydrochloric acid (2 mol/l).
2. Magnesium powder.
3. Chromotropic acid (solid).
4. Concentrated sulfuric acid (relative density 1.83).

Method

1. Add 0.1 ml of dilute hydrochloric acid to 0.1 ml of test solution and vortex-mix for 5 seconds.

2. Slowly add about 100 mg of magnesium powder until the evolution of gas ceases.
3. Add about 100 mg of chromotropic acid and vortex-mix for 5 seconds.
4. **Carefully** add 1.5 ml of concentrated sulfuric acid and heat in a water-bath at 60 °C for 10 minutes.

Results

A purple-violet colour indicates the presence of formates or formic acid. Formaldehyde reacts without prior reduction.

Sensitivity

Formate, 50 mg/l.

Clinical interpretation

Formic acid is very corrosive to tissues, and ingestion may cause burning and ulceration of the mouth and throat, corrosion of the glottis, oesophagus and stomach, metabolic acidosis, intravascular haemolysis, disseminated intravascular coagulation, circulatory collapse and renal and respiratory failure. Treatment is symptomatic and supportive.

6.53 Glutethimide

2-Ethyl-2-phenylglutarimide; $C_{13}H_{15}NO_2$; relative molecular mass, 217

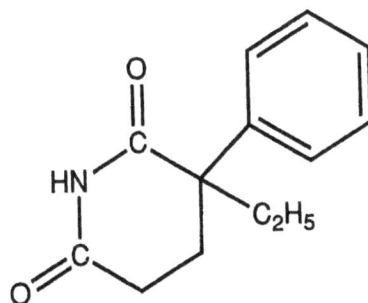

Glutethimide is a nonbarbiturate hypnotic which is now little used because of the risk of toxicity. The estimated minimum lethal dose of glutethimide in an adult is 5 g. Glutethimide forms a number of metabolites in humans, many of which are excreted in urine. Less than 2% of a dose is excreted unchanged.

There is no simple qualitative test for glutethimide, but this compound and its metabolites can be detected and identified by thin-layer chromatography of an acidic solvent extract of urine (see section 5.2.3).

Glutethimide is unstable at pH 11 and above, and the rapid decline in absorbance at 240 nm observed when a solution containing this compound is treated with concentrated ammonium hydroxide (see section 6.9) provides a further means of identification.

Clinical interpretation

Acute ingestion of glutethimide may cause dilated and unreactive pupils, hypotension, severe metabolic acidosis, coma, cerebral oedema, papilloedema and acute respiratory failure. Treatment is generally symptomatic and supportive. Charcoal haemoperfusion may be indicated in severe cases.

6.54 Glyceryl trinitrate

Trinitroglycerin; nitroglycerin; propane-1,2,3-triol trinitrate; $C_3H_5N_3O_9$; relative molecular mass, 227

Glyceryl trinitrate is used as a vasodilator in the treatment of angina and as an explosive in dynamite. Other organic nitro compounds (amyl nitrite, butyl nitrite) are also vasodilators and are commonly abused. The estimated minimum lethal dose of glyceryl trinitrate in an adult is 2 g. Glyceryl trinitrate is rapidly metabolized *in vivo* to dinitrates and mononitrates. About 20% of a sublingual dose is excreted in urine in 24 hours, mainly as the mononitrate.

> **Take care** — glyceryl trinitrate explodes on rapid heating or impact and is unsafe in alcoholic solution.

Qualitative test

Applicable to stomach contents and scene residues.

Reagents

1. Diphenylamine (10 ml/l) in concentrated sulfuric acid (relative density 1.83).
2. Silica gel thin-layer chromatography plate (5 × 20 cm, 20 μm average particle size; see section 4.4.1).

Standard

Aqueous glyceryl trinitrate (20 mg/l).

Method

1. Add 4 ml of chloroform:propan-2-ol (9:1) to 1 ml of sample or standard in a glass-stoppered test-tube.
2. Vortex-mix for 1 minute, allow to stand for 1 minute and discard the upper (aqueous) layer.
3. Filter the chloroform extract through phase-separating filter-paper into a clean tube and evaporate to dryness without heating under a stream of compressed air or nitrogen.

Thin-layer chromatography

1. Reconstitute the extract in 100 μl of chloroform and spot 20 μl of the sample and standard extracts on adjacent columns of the plate.
2. Develop the chromatogram in chloroform:acetone (4:1) (10-cm run, saturated tanks, see section 4.4.3).
3. Allow to dry and spray with diphenylamine solution.

Results

Glyceryl trinitrate (hR_f 0.71) gives a blue spot on a white background.

Sensitivity

Glyceryl trinitrate, 5 mg/l.

Clinical interpretation

Many of the signs and symptoms of poisoning with glyceryl trinitrate and other organic nitrates and nitrites are similar to those observed with inorganic nitrates and nitrites. Thus acute poisoning with organic nitrates or nitrites may cause headache, nausea, vomiting, diarrhoea, abdominal pain, flushing, dizziness, confusion, hypotension, collapse, coma and convulsions. Methaemoglobinaemia can be produced and this may be indicated by dark chocolate-coloured blood (see section 3.2.2). Blood methaemoglobin can be measured, but is unstable and the use of stored samples is unreliable. Treatment is symptomatic and supportive.

6.55 Haloperidol

4-[4-(4-Chlorophenyl)-4-hydroxypiperidino]-4′-fluorobutyrophenone; $C_{21}H_{23}ClFNO_2$; relative molecular mass, 376

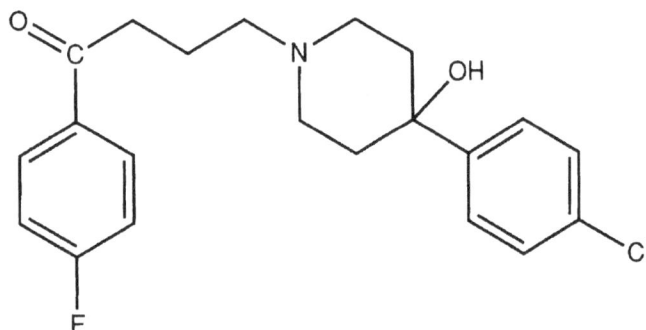

Haloperidol is a neuroleptic used orally or parenterally to treat schizophrenia and a variety of other disorders. Haloperidol is slowly excreted in urine following oral dosage, about 40% being eliminated within 5 days, about 1% as unchanged drug.

There is no simple qualitative test for haloperidol, but it can be detected and identified by thin-layer chromatography of a basic solvent extract of stomach contents or scene residues (see section 5.2.3). Urinary concentrations are often below the limit of detection of this method, even after overdosage.

Clinical interpretation

Acute overdosage with haloperidol and other butyrophenones may cause drowsiness, hypotension, dystonic reactions and akathisia. Treatment is largely symptomatic and supportive.

6.56 Hydroxybenzonitrile herbicides

The hydroxybenzonitriles encountered most commonly are bromoxynil (3,5-dibromo-4-hydroxybenzonitrile; $C_7H_3Br_2NO$; relative molecular mass, 277) and ioxynil (3,5-diiodo-4-hydroxybenzonitrile; $C_7H_3I_2NO$; relative molecular mass, 371).

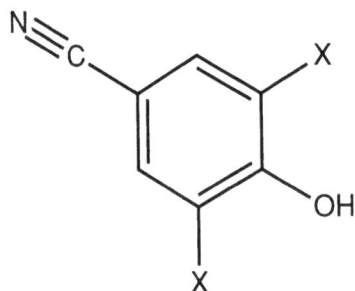

These compounds are contact herbicides with some systemic activity, and are widely used on cereal crops. Both bromoxynil and ioxynil uncouple oxidative phosphorylation so that poisoning with these compounds follows a similar course to that with other uncouplers such as the dinitrophenol pesticides and pentachlorophenol, and may follow occupational exposure as well as oral ingestion.

There are no simple tests for these compounds. However, both bromoxynil and ioxynil show high ultraviolet absorbance at 255 nm, and this forms the basis of the quantitative assay outlined below.

Quantitative assay

Applicable to plasma or serum (1.0 ml).

Reagent

Aqueous trichloroacetic acid (10 g/l).

Standards

Solutions containing either compound at concentrations of 20, 50, 100, 200 and 400 mg/l in blank human plasma.

Method

1. Add 1 ml of trichloroacetic acid solution to 1 ml of sample or standard in a 10-ml test-tube fitted with a ground-glass stopper.
2. Add 5 ml of methyl tertiary-butyl ether, vortex-mix for 30 seconds and centrifuge for 5 minutes.
3. Remove the upper (ether) layer and filter through phase-separating filter-paper into a clean tube.
4. Measure the absorbance at 255 nm against a blank plasma extract (see section 4.5.2).

Results

Construct a calibration graph of absorbance against hydroxybenzonitrile concentration in the calibration standards and calculate the hydroxybenzonitrile concentration in the sample. Care must be taken to minimize loss of methyl tertiary-butyl ether by evaporation before the absorption of the extract is measured.

Chlorophenoxy herbicides and other compounds that are highly soluble in water do not interfere. However, if a scanning spectrophotometer is available, comparison of the absorption spectra of sample and standard extracts at 220–300 nm may reveal the presence of other interfering compounds (see section 4.5.2).

Sensitivity

Bromoxynil or ioxynil, 20 mg/l.

Clinical interpretation

Absorption of bromoxynil and ioxynil may give rise to fatigue, irritability, excessive sweating, hyperthermia, tachycardia, vomiting and thirst, which may be followed by exhaustion and cardiorespiratory arrest. However, there is no characteristic staining of the skin as with the dinitrophenol pesticides. Treatment is largely symptomatic and supportive. As with the chlorophenoxy herbicides, alkalinization may protect against the systemic toxicity of these compounds. Plasma concentrations of either compound greater than 20 mg/l may be associated with clinical features of toxicity.

6.57 Hypochlorites

Hypochlorites such as sodium hypochlorite (NaOCl) and calcium hypochlorite (bleaching powder, chlorinated lime, $Ca(OCl)_2$) are widely used in bleach and disinfectant solutions. Domestic bleach is a 30–60 g/l aqueous solution of sodium hypochlorite, but higher concentrations (200 g/l) may be used, for example, to chlorinate swimming-pools.

Hypochlorites are strong oxidizing agents, and the test given below will also detect compounds with similar properties, such as bromates, chlorates, iodates, nitrates, and nitrites.

Qualitative test

Applicable to stomach contents and scene residues.

Reagent

Diphenylamine (10 g/l) in concentrated sulfuric acid (relative density 1.83).

Method

1. Filter, if necessary, 5 ml of stomach contents into a 10-ml glass tube.
2. Place 0.5 ml of filtrate or scene residue in a clean tube and **slowly** add 0.5 ml of diphenylamine solution down the side of the tube so that it forms a layer under the sample.

Results

A true positive is indicated by a strong blue colour which develops immediately at the junction of the two layers. A light blue colour will be given by most samples of stomach contents owing to the presence of organic material. As all strong oxidizing agents are rapidly reduced in biological samples, the test should be performed as soon as possible after receipt of the sample.

In contrast to other strong oxidizing agents, hypochlorites tend to evolve noxious green chlorine gas (**take care**) when treated with concentrated sulfuric acid, and this is a further diagnostic feature.

Sensitivity

Hypochlorite, 10 mg/l.

Confirmatory tests

Applicable to stomach contents and scene residues.

1. *Lead acetate test*

Reagents

1. Glacial acetic acid.
2. Aqueous lead acetate solution (50 g/l).

Method

1. Add acetic acid drop by drop to 1 ml of test solution to give a final pH of about 6 (universal indicator paper).
2. Add 0.5 ml of lead acetate solution and boil for 2–3 minutes.

Results

A brown precipitate confirms hypochlorite. Sulfides give an immediate brown/black precipitate with lead acetate solution.

Sensitivity

Hypochlorite, 10 mg/l.

2. *Potassium iodide/starch test*

Reagents

1. Aqueous potassium iodide solution (100 g/l).
2. Glacial acetic acid.
3. Starch (solid).

Method

1. Add 0.1 ml of test solution to 0.1 ml of acetic acid and then add 0.1 ml of potassium iodide solution.
2. Mix and add about 20 mg of starch.

Results

A blue colour confirms hypochlorite.

Sensitivity
Hypochlorite, 10 mg/l.

Clinical interpretation
Ingestion of hypochlorites may lead to the formation of hypochlorous acid by reaction with gastric acid, and this in turn may release free chlorine which may be inhaled. Features of poisoning with hypochlorites therefore include nausea, vomiting, diarrhoea, abdominal pain, confusion, hypotension, coma and pulmonary oedema. Irritation and corrosion of the mucous membranes, and oesophageal and gastric perforation may also occur, especially with more concentrated formulations. Treatment is symptomatic and supportive.

6.58 Imipramine

3-(10,11-Dihydro-5*H*-dibenz[*b,f*]azepin-5-yl)-*N,N*-dimethyl-propylamine; $C_{19}H_{24}N_2$; relative molecular mass, 280

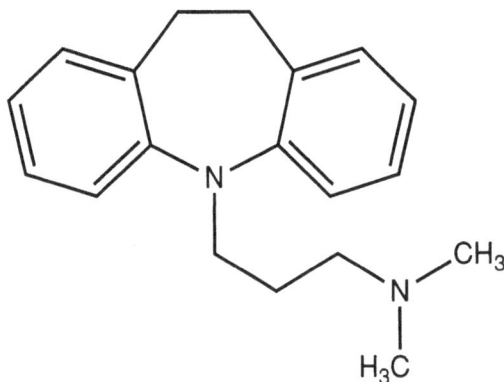

Imipramine is a widely used tricyclic antidepressant; it is metabolized by *N*-demethylation to desipramine, which is also used as an antidepressant in its own right. Trimipramine and clomipramine are analogues of imipramine.

The test described below (Forrest test) is based on the reaction of these compounds with acidified potassium dichromate solution.

Qualitative test
Applicable to urine, stomach contents and scene residues.

Reagent

Forrest reagent. Mix 25 ml of aqueous potassium dichromate solution (2 g/l) with 25 ml of aqueous sulfuric acid (300 ml/l), 25 ml of aqueous perchloric acid (200 g/kg) and 25 ml of aqueous nitric acid (500 ml/l).

Method

Add 1 ml of Forrest reagent to 0.5 ml of urine and vortex-mix for 5 seconds.

Results

A yellow-green colour deepening through dark green to blue indicates the presence of imipramine, desipramine, trimipramine or clomipramine. Phenothiazines may interfere and the FPN test for these latter compounds should also be performed (see section 6.91).

When applied to urine, this test will detect only acute overdosage. As with other tricyclic antidepressants, such as amitriptyline, greater sensitivity and selectivity can be obtained by thin-layer chromatography of a basic urine extract (see section 5.2.3), which should always be performed if possible.

Sensitivity

Imipramine, 25 mg/l.

Clinical interpretation

Acute poisoning with tricyclic antidepressants, such as imipramine, may be associated with dilated pupils, hypothermia, cardiac arrhythmias, respiratory depression, convulsions, coma and cardiorespiratory arrest. Urinary retention is also a feature of poisoning with these compounds, and this may delay procurement of an appropriate specimen for analysis.

Treatment is generally symptomatic and supportive. The use of antiarrhythmic agents is generally avoided, but alkalinization using sodium bicarbonate is sometimes employed. Quantitative measurements in blood are not normally required in management.

6.59 Iodates

Iodates such as potassium iodate (KIO_3) and sodium iodate ($NaIO_3$) are used as disinfectants, food additives, dietary supplements and chemical reagents. Iodates are strong oxidizing agents, and the test given below will also detect compounds with similar properties, such as bromates, chlorates, hypochlorites, nitrates and nitrites.

Qualitative test

Applicable to stomach contents and scene residues.

Reagent

Diphenylamine (10 g/l) in concentrated sulfuric acid (relative density 1.83).

Method

1. Filter, if necessary, 5 ml of stomach contents into a 10-ml glass tube.
2. Place 0.5 ml of filtrate or scene residue in a clean tube and **slowly** add 0.5 ml of diphenylamine solution down the side of the tube so that it forms a layer under the sample.

Results

A true positive is indicated by a strong blue colour which develops immediately at the junction of the two layers. A light blue colour will be given by most samples of stomach contents owing to the presence of organic material. As all strong oxidizing agents are rapidly reduced in biological samples, the test should be performed as soon as possible after receipt of the sample.

Sensitivity

Iodate, 1 mg/l.

Confirmatory test

Applicable to stomach contents and scene residues.

Reagents

1. Aqueous acetic acid (50 ml/l).
2. Aqueous starch solution (10 g/l, freshly prepared).
3. Aqueous potassium thiocyanate solution (50 g/l).

Method

1. To 0.1 ml of starch solution add 0.3 ml of purified water and 0.1 ml of potassium thiocyanate solution.
2. Mix well and add 0.1 ml of test solution acidified with 0.1 ml of acetic acid solution.

Results

A blue colour is specific for iodate. Iodate also reacts like chloride in the confirmatory test for bromates (see section 6.14).

Sensitivity

Iodate, 100 mg/l.

Clinical interpretation

Acute poisoning with iodates may cause nausea, vomiting, diarrhoea, abdominal pain, confusion, coma and convulsions. Methaemoglobinaemia is often produced and this may be indicated by dark chocolate-coloured blood (see section 3.2.2). Blood methaemoglobin can be measured, but is unstable and the use of stored samples is unreliable. Treatment is symptomatic and supportive.

6.60 Iodine and iodide

Iodine (I_2) is one of the oldest antiseptics in medicine. It is used topically as a solution in ethanol (tincture) containing elemental iodine together with potassium iodide (KI) or sodium iodide (NaI), which enhances the solubility of iodine itself by forming polyiodide ion. Potassium iodide and sodium iodide are themselves used as dietary supplements and in photography, but are relatively innocuous in comparison with iodine.

When iodine is applied to the skin or mucous membranes it is absorbed as iodide. The qualitative test given below serves to indicate the presence of inorganic iodides or bromides and the appropriate confirmatory tests must then be used.

Qualitative test

Applicable to urine, stomach contents and scene residues.

Reagents

1. Aqueous nitric acid (2 mol/l).
2. Aqueous silver nitrate solution (10 g/l).
3. Concentrated ammonium hydroxide (relative density 0.88).

Method

1. Add 0.1 ml of nitric acid to 1 ml of clear test solution, mix and add 0.1 ml of silver nitrate solution.
2. Centrifuge to isolate any significant precipitate and treat with 0.1 ml of ammonium hydroxide solution.

Results

A white precipitate soluble in ammonium hydroxide indicates chloride, an off-white precipitate sparingly soluble in ammonium hydroxide indicates bromide, and a creamy-yellow, insoluble precipitate indicates iodide.

Sensitivity

Iodide, 100 mg/l.

Confirmatory test

Applicable to urine, stomach contents and scene residues.

Reagents

1. Aqueous hydrochloric acid (2 mol/l).
2. Starch (solid).
3. Sodium nitrite solution (100 g/l, freshly prepared).

Method

Vortex-mix 0.1 ml of test solution, about 20 mg of starch, 0.1 ml of dilute hydrochloric acid and 0.1 ml of sodium nitrite solution in a test-tube.

Results

A blue colour confirms iodide.

Sensitivity

Iodide, 100 mg/l.

Clinical interpretation

Acute poisoning with iodine solutions may cause corrosion of the mucous membranes of the mouth, oesophagus and stomach, vomiting, diarrhoea and abdominal pain. In severe cases, delirium, coma, circulatory collapse and acute renal failure may ensue. Absorption of as little as 2–4 g of free iodine may cause death. Treatment is generally symptomatic and supportive. Starch may be administered to adsorb orally ingested iodine.

Acute ingestion of iodide salts may cause angioedema, swelling of the larynx and cutaneous haemorrhages. However, as with bromides, signs of toxicity are more likely to occur with chronic poisoning, and include the presence of a burning sensation in the mouth and throat, metallic taste, sore teeth and gums, hypersalivation, headache, pulmonary oedema, enlargement of the parotid and submaxillary glands, anorexia, diarrhoea, fever and depression. Treatment is symptomatic and supportive.

6.61 Iron

Ferrous (iron II) salts are used in the treatment of iron deficiency anaemia and ferric (iron III) salts, which are more toxic, have been used as abortifacients. The minimum lethal dose of ferrous sulfate in an adult is of the order of 30 g, but 1 g may be dangerous in an infant. A green or blue colour in vomit or stomach contents suggests the presence of iron or copper salts.

The qualitative test given below can be used to differentiate between ferrous and ferric iron and other metals, while the quantitative assay can be used to measure serum iron. It is very important to avoid contamination when collecting blood for the measurement of serum iron concentrations; vigorous discharge of the sample through the syringe needle can cause sufficient haemolysis to invalidate the assay.

Qualitative test

Applicable to stomach contents and scene residues.

Reagents

1. Aqueous hydrochloric acid (2 mol/l).
2. Aqueous potassium ferricyanide solution (10 g/l).
3. Aqueous potassium ferrocyanide solution (10 g/l).

Method

1. To 0.1 ml of sample add 0.1 ml of dilute hydrochloric acid and 0.05 ml of potassium ferricyanide solution and vortex-mix for 5 seconds.
2. To a further 0.1 ml of sample add 0.1 ml of dilute hydrochloric acid and 0.05 ml of potassium ferrocyanide solution, and vortex-mix for 5 seconds.
3. Leave for 5 minutes at ambient temperature and centrifuge for 5 minutes.

Results

Deep blue precipitates with potassium ferricyanide (step 1) and potassium ferrocyanide (step 2) indicate the presence of ferrous and ferric iron, respectively.

Sensitivity

Ferrous or ferric iron, 10 mg/l.

Quantitative assay

Applicable to unhaemolysed serum (2 ml).

Reagents

1. Aqueous sodium sulfite solution (0.1 mol/l, freshly prepared).
2. 2,2'-Bipyridyl (1 g/l) in aqueous acetic acid (30 ml/l).
3. Aqueous hydrochloric acid (0.005 mol/l).

Standards

Prepare aqueous solutions containing ferrous ion concentrations of 1.0, 2.0, 5.0 and 10.0 mg/l by dilution of ferrous ammonium sulfate solution (1.00 g of ferrous iron per litre) with dilute hydrochloric acid.

Method

1. Mix 2 ml of sample, 2 ml of sodium sulfite solution and 2 ml of 2,2'-bipyridyl solution in a 10-ml centrifuge tube with a ground-glass neck.
2. Heat in a boiling water-bath for 5 minutes, cool and add 1 ml of chloroform.
3. Stopper, rotary-mix for 5 minutes and then centrifuge for 5 minutes.
4. If an emulsion forms, vortex-mix for 30 seconds and repeat the centrifugation.
5. Remove the chloroform extract, filter through phase-separating filter-paper and measure the absorbance of the extract at 520 nm against a reagent blank (see section 4.5.2).

Results

Construct a calibration graph of absorbance against ferrous iron concentration in the calibration standards and calculate the iron concentration in the sample.

This method should not be used if chelating agents such as deferoxamine have been given before the specimen was obtained, since the result may not be reliable.

Sensitivity

Iron, 0.5 mg/l.

Clinical interpretation

Acute poisoning with iron salts is extremely dangerous, especially in young children. The absorbed iron may rapidly exceed the binding capacity of transferrin so that free iron accumulates in the blood. Rapid necrosis of the gastrointestinal mucosa may occur with haemorrhage and loss of electrolytes and fluid. Treatment may include chelation therapy with deferoxamine, given intravenously or orally (see Table 6).

Normal serum iron concentrations are less than 1.8 mg/l (34 μmol/l). Serious toxicity may occur at concentrations above 5 mg/l (90 μmol/l) in children or above 8 mg/l (145 μmol/l) in adults. The serum iron concentration should be measured before and during chelation therapy, both to confirm the need for such treatment and to monitor efficacy.

6.62 Isoniazid

Isonicotinic acid hydrazide; INAH; INH; isonicotinohydrazide; $C_6H_7N_3O$; relative molecular mass, 137

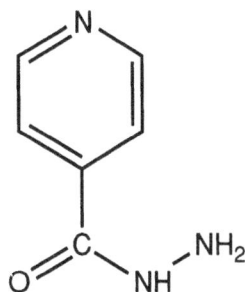

Isoniazid is used in the treatment of tuberculosis. The principal metabolic reaction is acetylation, but other reactions include hydrolysis, conjugation with glycine and N-methylation. Up to 70% of a dose is excreted in urine, largely as metabolites. Serious toxicity may occur in adults with doses of 3 g.

The colorimetric procedure given below can be used to measure the plasma isoniazid concentration if overdosage with this drug is suspected.

Quantitative assay
Applicable to plasma or serum (2 ml).

Reagents
1. Aqueous metaphosphoric acid (200 g/l).
2. Aqueous acetic acid (2 mol/l).
3. Sodium nitroprusside reagent. Mix 25 ml of aqueous sodium nitroprusside (20 g/l) with 25 ml of aqueous sodium hydroxide (4 mol/l), freshly prepared.

Standards
Standard solutions containing isoniazid concentrations of 5, 10, 20 and 50 mg/l in blank plasma.

Method

1. Add 4 ml of purified water to 2 ml of sample and add 2 ml of dilute metaphosphoric acid.
2. Vortex-mix for 30 seconds and allow to stand for 10 minutes.
3. Centrifuge for 5 minutes and transfer 4 ml of the supernatant to a clean tube.
4. Add 2 ml of dilute acetic acid, 2 ml of sodium nitroprusside reagent and vortex-mix for 5 seconds.
5. Allow to stand for 2 minutes and measure the absorbance at 440 nm against a plasma blank (see section 4.5.2).

Results

Prepare a calibration graph by analysis of the standard isoniazid solutions and calculate the isoniazid concentration in the sample. Specimens containing isoniazid at concentrations greater than 50 mg/l should be diluted with blank plasma and re-analysed.

Related drugs such as iproniazid and pyrazinamide interfere in this test. 4-Aminosalicylate also interferes, but only if present at a high concentration.

Sensitivity

Isoniazid, 5 mg/l.

Clinical interpretation

Overdosage with isoniazid may cause nausea, vomiting, dilated pupils, hypotension, hyperglycaemia, oliguria, metabolic acidosis, coma, convulsions, and circulatory and respiratory failure. Treatment is generally symptomatic and supportive, although intravenous administration of pyridoxine (vitamin B_6) is indicated in severe cases (see Table 4).

The plasma isoniazid concentrations attained during therapy are normally less than 10 mg/l. Toxicity has been associated with plasma concentrations greater than 20 mg/l, and blood concentrations of up to 150 mg/l have been reported in fatalities.

6.63 Laxatives

Laxatives are sometimes abused by patients with eating disorders such as bulimia or anorexia nervosa. Some commonly encountered laxatives are listed in Table 28. Bisacodyl, dantron and phenolphthalein are synthetic compounds, while rhein is a common constituent of many laxatives of vegetable origin (senna, cascara, frangula and rhubarb root).

The test given below, which involves thin-layer chromatography of a solvent extract of a hydrolysed urine specimen, is especially useful in differentiating between diarrhoea due to microbial infection or food allergy and that due to self-medication with laxatives.

Table 28. Some common laxatives

Compound	Chemical name	Relative molecular mass
Bisacodyl	4,4'-(2-Pyridylmethylene)di(phenyl acetate)	361
Dantron	1,8-Dihydroxyanthraquinone	240
Phenolphthalein	3,3-Bis(4-hydroxyphenyl)phthalide	318
Rhein	9,10-Dihydro-4,5-dihydroxy-9,10-dioxo-2-anthracene carboxylic acid	284

Qualitative test

Applicable to urine.

Reagents

1. Aqueous sodium hydroxide solution (6 mol/l).
2. Sodium acetate buffer. Adjust 300 g/l of sodium acetate dihydrate to pH 5 with glacial acetic acid.
3. Ketodase solution (β-glucuronidase 5000 units/ml).
4. Chloroform:propan-2-ol (9:1)
5. *m*-Xylene:isopropylacetone:methanol (10:10:1) (XIAM).
6. *n*-Hexane:toluene:glacial acetic acid (3:1:1) (HTAA).
7. Silica gel thin-layer chromatography plates (20 × 20 cm, 20 μm average particle size, see section 4.4.1).

Standards

1. Bisacodyl. Dissolve 2 mg in 10 ml of methanol. Add 100 μl of sodium hydroxide solution and heat on a water-bath for 30 minutes at 70 °C to prepare the monohydroxy and dihydroxy analogues.
2. Dantron (2 mg in 10 ml of chloroform).
3. Phenolphthalein (2 mg in 200 μl of methanol and 10 ml of chloroform).
4. Rhein (2 mg in 10 ml of chloroform).

   These solutions are stable for at least 2 months if stored in stoppered tubes at 4 °C.

Method

1. To 20 ml of urine add 1 ml of ketodase and 2 ml of sodium acetate buffer.
2. Incubate in a water-bath for 2 hours at 60 °C.
3. Cool and add 25 ml of chloroform:propan-2-ol (9:1).
4. Vortex-mix for 5 minutes, centrifuge for 5 minutes and remove the upper, aqueous layer by aspiration.

5. Evaporate the organic extract to dryness under a stream of compressed air or, preferably, nitrogen at 40 °C.

Thin-layer chromatography

1. Reconstitute the extract in 100 μl of chloroform.
2. Spot 10 μl of the reference solutions and 3 μl and 10 μl of the reconstituted extract on to each of two plates.
3. Develop plate 1 in XIAM and plate 2 in HTAA (10-cm run, saturated tanks, see section 4.4.3).
4. Inspect under ultraviolet light at 366 nm and mark the outline of the spots with a pencil.
5. Spray each plate with sodium hydroxide solution.

Results

The thin-layer chromatography characteristics of the compounds studied are given in Table 29. This method will detect a single dose of the named laxatives up to about 36 hours after ingestion.

Note that bisacodyl is only detected after hydrolysis as a dihydroxy compound and as a hydroxylated metabolite at a lower hR_f value on the XIAM plate. Both of these compounds give a purple colour with the sodium hydroxide spray.

Sensitivity

Each laxative, about 0.2 mg/l.

Clinical interpretation

Chronic ingestion of laxatives may lead to diarrhoea, hypokalaemia and large bowel dilatation, while additional problems, such as skin disorders (with phenolphthalein), may occur in certain patients.

Table 29. **Thin-layer chromatography of laxatives: hR_f values and colours**

Compound	hR_f		Ultra-violet (366 nm)	Sodium hydroxide
	XIAM	HTAA		
Rhein	02	19	Orange	Red
Bisacodyl metabolite	17	—	—	Purple/grey
Dihydroxybisacodyl	21	—	—	Red/purple
Monohydroxybisacodyl	26	—	—	Red/purple
Bisacodyl	30	—	—	Red/purple
Phenolphthalein	32	05	—	Red
Dantron	45	27	Orange	Yellow

6.64 Lead

Lead (Pb) and lead compounds have a number of industrial uses ranging from paint additives to solder, batteries and building materials. Well known insoluble lead compounds include red lead (Pb_3O_4) and white lead (basic lead carbonate, $PbCO_3.Pb(OH)_2$). The most important soluble salts of lead are lead nitrate ($Pb(NO_3)_2$) and lead acetate ($Pb(CH_3COO)_2$). This latter compound is also known as sugar of lead because of its sweet taste. Organic lead compounds, such as tetraethyl lead, are still used as antiknock agents in petrol.

There is no simple qualitative test for lead that can be carried out on biological samples. However, physical and chemical tests on materials suspected of containing lead may be useful. Lead compounds will usually sink to the bottom when sprinkled into a glass of water, and this may be useful in the examination of paint flakes or cosmetics, such as surma (an Asian preparation often containing antimony or lead). It should be borne in mind that finely divided lead compounds may float on the surface as a result of the surface tension of the water.

Qualitative test

Applicable to stomach contents and scene residues.

Reagents

1. Sodium tartrate buffer, pH 2.8. Mix sodium bitartate (19 g/l) and tartaric acid (15 g/l) in purified water.
2. Aqueous sodium rhodizonate solution (10 g/l).

Method

1. Add 0.1 ml of sodium tartrate buffer to 0.1 ml of test solution and vortex-mix for 5 seconds.
2. Spot 50 μl of acidified solution on to phase-separating filter-paper and add 50 μl of sodium rhodizonate solution.

Results

Lead salts give a purple colour in this test. However, the test is not specific: barium salts give a brown colour and a number of other metals also give coloured complexes.

Sensitivity

Lead, 2 mg/l.

Clinical interpretation

The acute ingestion of soluble lead salts may cause severe colicky pain with constipation or diarrhoea. Chronic lead poisoning is more common and additional symptoms include fatigue, anaemia and joint weakness

161

and pain. Lead poisoning in young children may cause coma and encephalopathy. Treatment may include chelation therapy.

In the absence of facilities for the accurate measurement of lead concentration in blood, a diagnosis of lead poisoning is best made from a careful evaluation of the history and clinical presentation. Nonspecific signs that may indicate a diagnosis of chronic lead poisoning include basophilic stippling of red cells, a blue gum line and wrist drop. Specialized clinical chemical tests that may also assist in diagnosis include red-cell zinc protoporphyrin concentration and urinary δ-amino-laevulinic acid excretion, but again suitable facilities may not be available.

6.65 Lidocaine

Lignocaine; 2-diethylaminoaceto-2',6'-xylidide; $C_{14}H_{22}N_2O$; relative molecular mass, 234

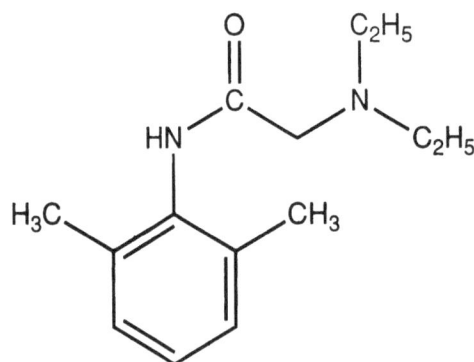

Lidocaine is used as a local anaesthetic and is commonly found in lubricant gels for use with urinary catheters. It is also used as an antiarrhythmic but is only effective when given intravenously, since it undergoes extensive first-pass metabolism. Metabolic pathways include N-dealkylation, hydroxylation, amide hydrolysis and glucuronide formation; only some 3% of an oral dose is excreted unchanged in urine. The fatal oral dose of lidocaine is about 25 g in an adult.

Lidocaine is often found in urine and other samples from oisoned patients, sometimes in very high concentrations. This usually results from topical use of a lubricant gel containing lidocaine. Metabolites may also occur in urine following topical use of lidocaine.

There is no simple qualitative test for lidocaine, but it can be detected and identified by thin-layer chromatography of a basic solvent extract of urine, stomach contents or scene residues (see section 5.2.3).

Clinical interpretation

Acute poisoning with lidocaine may cause confusion, paraesthesia, hypotension, coma, convulsions and circulatory collapse. Treatment is symptomatic and supportive.

6.66 Lithium

Lithium (Li) salts have a number of industrial uses, and lithium carbonate (Li_2CO_3; relative molecular mass, 74) and lithium citrate ($C_6H_5Li_3O_7 \cdot 4H_2O$; relative molecular mass, 282) are widely used in the treatment of depression and mania. Lithium is excreted in urine, but the plasma half-life is dependent on the duration of therapy, among other factors. In therapy, 2 g of lithium carbonate may be given daily for 5–7 days, but this is normally reduced to 0.6–1.2 g/day thereafter. Survival has followed the acute ingestion of 22 g of lithium carbonate, although this is unusual.

There is no simple method for the measurement of lithium in biological specimens. The test given below can be used to indicate the presence of lithium salts in samples which contain relatively high concentrations of this element.

Qualitative test
Applicable to scene residues.

Reagents

1. Concentrated hydrochloric acid (relative density 1.18).
2. Platinum wire.

Method

1. Dip the end of the platinum wire in the concentrated acid.
2. Dip the moistened end of the wire into the test material.
3. Place the material in the hot part of the flame of a microburner.

Results

A crimson red flame denotes the presence of lithium salts. However, calcium and strontium salts also give red flames, while high concentrations of sodium (yellow flame) can mask other colours.

Sensitivity
Lithium, 50 mg/l.

Clinical interpretation

Acute poisoning with lithium salts can cause nausea, vomiting, apathy, drowsiness, tremor, ataxia and muscular rigidity, with coma, convulsions and death in severe cases. Overdosage with lithium tends to be more serious in patients on chronic lithium therapy, since tissue sites are saturated and lithium accumulates in plasma. Treatment is symptomatic and supportive, but peritoneal dialysis or haemodialysis may be indicated in severe cases (see section 2.2.3).

6.67 Meprobamate

2-Methyl-2-*iso*-propylpropane-1,3-diol dicarbamate; $C_9H_{18}N_2O_4$; relative molecular mass, 218

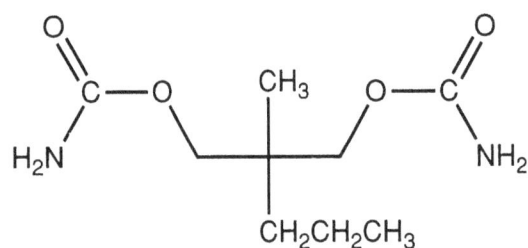

Meprobamate is a sedative and tranquillizer. Metabolites include meprobamate *N*-oxide and 2-hydroxypropylmeprobamate. About 90% of a dose is excreted in urine, 15% as unchanged drug. The estimated minimum lethal dose in an adult is 12 g, but recovery has occurred after much larger doses.

The qualitative test described here is based on a general reaction of carbamates with furfuraldehyde in the presence of hydrogen chloride. The confirmatory test is also applicable to urine, and is based on solvent extraction followed by thin-layer chromatography of the concentrated extract.

Qualitative test

Applicable to stomach contents and scene residues.

Reagents

1. Aqueous hydrochloric acid (2 mol/l).
2. Furfuraldehyde solution (100 ml/l) in methanol, freshly prepared.
3. Concentrated hydrochloric acid (relative density 1.18).

Method

1. Acidify 1 ml of sample with 0.5 ml of dilute hydrochloric acid, and extract with 4 ml of chloroform on a rotary mixer for 5 minutes.
2. Centrifuge in a bench centrifuge for 5 minutes, discard the upper, aqueous phase and filter the chloroform extract through phase-separating filter-paper into a clean tube.
3. Evaporate the extract to dryness under a stream of compressed air or nitrogen at 40 °C.
4. Dissolve the residue in 0.1 ml of methanol and apply a 10-mm diameter spot to filter-paper, and allow to dry.
5. Apply 0.1 ml of furfuraldehyde solution to the spot, and allow to dry.
6. Expose the paper to concentrated hydrochloric acid fumes for 5 minutes **in a fume cupboard**.

Results

Meprobamate gives a black spot. Other carbamates, such as the carbamate pesticides, interfere in this test.

Sensitivity

Meprobamate, 100 mg/l.

Confirmatory test

Applicable to urine, stomach contents and scene residues.

Reagents

1. Aqueous hydrochloric acid (1 mol/l).
2. Methanol : concentrated ammonium hydroxide (relative density 0.88) (100:1.5) (MA, see also section 6.73).
3. Furfuraldehyde (20 ml/l) in acetone, freshly prepared.
4. Concentrated sulfuric acid (relative density 1.83) solution (40 ml/l) in acetone, freshly prepared.
5. Van Urk reagent. Mix 1 g of *p*-dimethylaminobenzaldehyde in 100 ml of methanol with 10 ml of concentrated hydrochloric acid (relative density 1.18).
6. Silica gel thin-layer chromatography plates (10 × 20 cm, 20 μm average particle size, see section 4.4.1).

Standard

Meprobamate 1 g/l in chloroform.

Method

1. Add 1 ml of dilute hydrochloric acid and 10 ml of chloroform to 10 ml of urine in a 30-ml glass tube.

2. Rotary-mix for 5 minutes, centrifuge for 5 minutes and discard the upper, aqueous phase.
3. Transfer the lower, organic layer to a 15-ml tapered glass tube and evaporate to dryness in a water-bath at 60 °C under a stream of compressed air or nitrogen.

Thin-layer chromatography

1. Reconstitute the extract in 100 μl of chloroform and spot two portions of 50 μl of the extract and two portions of 10 μl of the meprobamate standard on to separate columns of the plate.
2. Develop (10-cm run) using MA (saturated tank, see section 4.4.3) and dry until no smell of ammonia remains.
3. Spray one pair of columns (sample and standard) sequentially with (*a*) furfuraldehyde solution and (*b*) sulfuric acid solution, and allow to dry.
4. Spray the second pair of columns with van Urk reagent.

Results

Meprobamate (hR$_f$, 10) gives a violet reaction with the furfuraldehyde/sulfuric acid spray, and a yellow colour with van Urk reagent. It may be necessary to redistill the furfuraldehyde, since this compound polymerizes on standing giving a brown discoloration. The sensitivity of the furfuraldehyde/sulfuric acid spray may be increased by gently heating the plate with a hair-drier after spraying.

Other carbamate drugs, such as carisoprodol, mebutamate and tybamate, may interfere in this test, but meprobamate is by far the most common compound encountered.

Sensitivity

Meprobamate, 10 mg/l.

Clinical interpretation

Acute meprobamate poisoning may cause hypotension, hypothermia, muscle weakness, nystagmus, acidosis, coma, respiratory depression, pulmonary oedema, acute renal failure and disseminated intravascular coagulation. Treatment is normally symptomatic and supportive.

6.68 Mercury

Mercury (Hg) and its inorganic salts are used in the manufacture of thermometers, felt, paints, explosives, lamps, electrical equipment and batteries. Diethyl mercury, dimethyl mercury and a variety of other mercury compounds, including inorganic mercurials, are used as fungicides, primarily on seeds and bulbs, and in lawn sands. Mercuric chloride ($HgCl_2$) is extremely toxic and ingestion of 1 g may prove fatal in an adult. As with antimony, arsenic and bismuth, mercury can be detected using the Reinsch test.

Qualitative test

Applicable to urine, stomach contents and scene residues. Reinsch test — see antimony monograph (section 6.5)

Results

Staining on the copper can be interpreted as follows:

purple black — antimony
dull black — arsenic
shiny black — bismuth
silver — mercury

Selenium and tellurium may also give dark deposits, while high concentrations of sulfur may give a speckled appearance to the copper.

Confirmatory test

Applicable to silver-stained foil from the Reinsch test.

Reagent

Copper (I) iodide suspension. Dissolve 5 g of copper (II) sulfate and 3 g of ferrous sulfate in 10 ml of purified water with continuous stirring and add 7 g of potassium iodide in 50 ml of water. Allow the copper (I) iodide precipitate to form, filter and wash with water. Transfer to a brown glass bottle as a suspension with the aid of a little water. This suspension is quite stable.

Method

Add 0.1 ml of copper (I) iodide suspension to a filter-paper, place the foil on the suspension, cover and leave for 1–12 hours.

Results

A salmon-pink colour indicates the presence of mercury. Positive results may be obtained within 1 hour, but with low concentrations, colour development may take up to 12 hours.

Sensitivity

Mercury, 5 mg/l.

Clinical interpretation

Elemental mercury is poorly absorbed from the gastrointestinal tract and is not considered toxic by this route. Mercury vapour is absorbed through the skin and lungs and may give rise to stomatitis, increased salivation, a metallic taste, diarrhoea, pneumonitis and renal failure. The ingestion of mercuric salts may cause severe gastric pain, vomiting, bloody diarrhoea and also renal failure, which is usually the cause of death. Organomercurials are concentrated in the central nervous system and produce ataxia, chorea and convulsions.

Treatment is symptomatic and supportive and may include chelation therapy. Mercury concentrations in blood and urine are good indicators of exposure, but only atomic absorption spectrophotometric methods of determination are reliable.

6.69 Methadone

($\pm$)-6-Dimethylamino-4,4-diphenylheptan-3-one; $C_{21}H_{27}NO$; relative molecular mass, 310

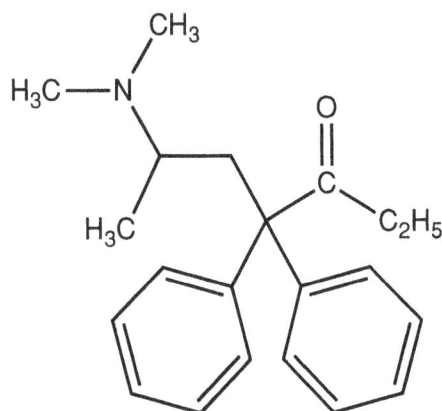

Methadone is a narcotic analgesic structurally related to dextropropoxyphene and is widely used in the treatment of opioid dependence. Methadone is metabolized largely by *N*-demethylation and hydroxylation. However, approximately 30% of an oral dose is excreted unchanged in urine. Plasma methadone concentrations attained on chronic (maintenance) therapy are very much higher than those associated with serious toxicity in patients not taking methadone chronically.

There is no simple qualitative test for methadone, but this compound and its metabolites can be detected and identified by thin-layer chromatography of a basic solvent extract of urine (see section 5.2.3).

Clinical interpretation

Acute overdosage with methadone may give rise to pin-point pupils, hypotension, hypothermia, coma, convulsions and pulmonary oedema. Death may ensue from profound respiratory depression. Naloxone rapidly reverses the central toxic effects of methadone (see section 2.2.2).

6.70 Methanol

Methyl alcohol; wood alcohol; CH_3OH; relative molecular mass, 32

Methanol is used as a general and laboratory solvent, and in antifreeze (often with ethylene glycol), windscreen washer additives and duplicating fluids. In an adult, death may follow the ingestion of 20–50 ml of methanol. Poisoning with industrial grades of ethanol (methylated spirit), which often contain methanol as a denaturant, also occurs, but is generally less serious than with methanol alone. This is because methanol toxicity results from its metabolism to formaldehyde and formate by alcohol dehydrogenase, a reaction inhibited by ethanol.

Qualitative test

Applicable to urine, stomach contents and scene residues.

Reagent

Potassium dichromate reagent. Potassium dichromate (25 g/l) in purified water : concentrated sulfuric acid (relative density 1.83) (1:1).

Method

1. Apply 50 µl of potassium dichromate reagent to a strip of glass-fibre filter-paper and insert the paper in the neck of a test-tube containing 1 ml of urine.
2. Lightly stopper the tube and place in a boiling water-bath for 2 minutes.

Results

A change in colour from orange to green indicates the presence of volatile reducing agents such as methanol. However, other such compounds, for example ethanol, metaldehyde, and paraldehyde, also react.

Sensitivity

Methanol, 50 mg/l.

Confirmatory test

Applicable to urine, stomach contents and scene residues.

Reagents

1. Potassium dichromate reagent. Potassium dichromate (25 g/l) in purified water : concentrated sulfuric acid (relative density 1.83) (1:1).
2. Concentrated sulfuric acid (relative density 1.83).
3. Chromotropic acid (solid).

Method

1. Add 0.1 ml of potassium dichromate reagent to 1 ml of urine and allow to stand at room temperature for 5 minutes.
2. Add 0.1 ml of ethanol and about 10 mg of chromotropic acid and **gently** add sulfuric acid down the side of the tube so that it forms a separate layer at the bottom.

Results

A violet colour at the junction of the two layers indicates the presence of methanol. Formaldehyde also gives a positive result in this test.

Sensitivity

Methanol, 50 mg/l.

Clinical interpretation

Acute methanol poisoning is characterized by delayed onset of coma, cyanosis, respiratory failure, marked metabolic acidosis, electrolyte imbalance, hyperglycaemia and blindness, which may be permanent. Treatment is aimed at correcting metabolic abnormalities, inhibiting methanol metabolism by giving ethanol and removing unchanged methanol by peritoneal dialysis or haemodialysis. Measurement of plasma ethanol concentrations can be useful in monitoring therapy with this compound (see section 6.46).

6.71 Methaqualone

2-Methyl-3-*o*-tolylquinazolin-4(3H)-one; $C_{16}H_{14}N_2O$; relative molecular mass, 250

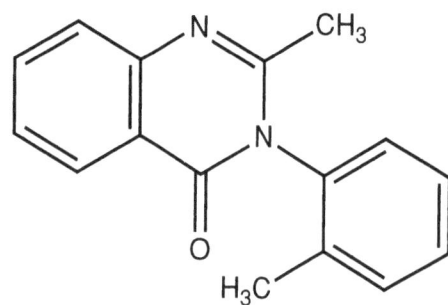

Methaqualone is a nonbarbiturate hypnotic, but is now little used because of the risk of toxicity. Metabolic pathways include aromatic hydroxylation, *N*-oxidation, and conjugation. Less than 2% of a dose is excreted unchanged. The estimated minimum lethal dose of methaqualone in an adult is 5 g.

There is no simple qualitative test for methaqualone, but it can be detected and identified by thin-layer chromatography of a basic solvent extract of urine, stomach contents or scene residues (see section 5.2.3).

Clinical interpretation

Acute methaqualone poisoning may cause hypertonia, myoclonus, papilloedema, tachycardia, pulmonary oedema, coma and convulsions. Treatment is generally symptomatic and supportive. Charcoal haemoperfusion may be indicated in severe cases.

6.72 Methyl bromide

Methyl bromide (CH_3Br) is used as a fumigant in ships' holds, grain silos and other large enclosed areas. Methyl bromide undergoes partial metabolism to give inorganic bromide *in vivo*. Since the concentrations of this ion encountered in methyl bromide poisoning are much lower than in serious poisoning with inorganic bromides, it is thought that methyl bromide itself is the primary toxin.

The qualitative test given below serves to indicate the presence of inorganic bromides or iodides, and the appropriate confirmatory test must then be used or blood bromide measured. There is no simple method for measuring unchanged methyl bromide.

Qualitative test

Applicable to urine. Detects inorganic bromide.

Reagents

1. Aqueous nitric acid (2 mol/l).
2. Aqueous silver nitrate solution (10 g/l).
3. Concentrated ammonium hydroxide (relative density 0.88).

Method

1. Add 0.1 ml of nitric acid to 1 ml of clear test solution, mix for 5 seconds and add 0.1 ml of silver nitrate solution.
2. Centrifuge to isolate any significant precipitate and treat with 0.1 ml of concentrated ammonium hydroxide.

Results

A white precipitate soluble in ammonium hydroxide indicates chloride, an off-white precipitate sparingly soluble in ammonium hydroxide indicates the presence of bromide and a creamy-yellow, insoluble precipitate indicates iodide.

Sensitivity

Bromide, 50 mg/l.

Confirmatory test

Applicable to urine. Detects inorganic bromide.

Reagents

1. Saturated fluorescein solution in aqueous acetic acid (600 ml/l).
2. Concentrated sulfuric acid (relative density 1.83).
3. Potassium permanganate (solid)

Method

1. Soak a strip of filter-paper in fluorescein solution.
2. Add about 50 mg of potassium permanganate to 2 ml of test solution in a 10-ml test-tube.
3. Add 0.2 ml of concentrated sulfuric acid and hold the fluorescein-impregnated filter-paper in the mouth of the tube.

Results

The bromide is oxidized to free bromine. This reacts with the yellow dye fluorescein to give eosin (tetrabromofluorescein) which has a pink/red colour.

Sensitivity

Bromide, 50 mg/l.

Quantitative assay

Applicable to plasma or serum (2 ml).

Reagents

1. Aqueous chloroauric acid. Dissolve 0.5 g of chloroauric acid (gold chloride, $HAuCl_4 \cdot xH_2O$) in 100 ml of purified water.
2. Aqueous trichloroacetic acid (200 g/l).

Standards

Dissolve 1.288 g of sodium bromide in 500 ml of purified water (bromide ion 2 g/l). Prepare serial dilutions in purified water containing bromide ion concentrations of 0.2, 0.4, 0.6, 0.8, 1.2 and 1.6 g/l.

Method

1. Add 6 ml of trichloroacetic acid solution to 2 ml of sample in a 10-ml test-tube, vortex-mix for 30 seconds and allow to stand for 15 minutes.
2. Centrifuge in a bench centrifuge for 5 minutes and filter the supernatant through phase-separating filter-paper into a clean tube.
3. Add 1 ml of chloroauric acid solution to 4 ml of the clear supernatant and vortex-mix for 5 seconds.
4. Record the absorbance at 440 nm against a purified water blank (see section 4.5.2).

Results

Construct a calibration graph of bromide concentration against absorbance by analysis of the standard bromide solutions, and calculate the concentration of bromide ion in the sample. The calibration is linear for concentrations from 25 mg/l to 2.5 g/l. This method is not reliable with specimens that may give turbid supernatants, e.g. postmortem samples.

Sensitivity

Bromide, 25 mg/l.

Clinical interpretation

Symptoms of poisoning due to methyl bromide often develop several hours after exposure and include confusion, dizziness, headache, nausea, vomiting, abdominal pain, blurred vision, hyporeflexia and paraesthesia. Coma and convulsions may occur in severe cases, and pulmonary oedema, jaundice and oliguria have also been described. Treatment is symptomatic and supportive.

Normal serum bromide concentrations are less than 10 mg/l. After the therapeutic administration of inorganic bromides, concentrations of up to 80 mg/l may be attained; toxicity is usually associated with concentrations greater than 500 mg/l. On the other hand, blood bromide concentrations of 90–400 mg/l have been reported in fatal methyl bromide poisoning.

6.73 Morphine

(4a*R*,5*S*,7a*R*,8*R*,9c*S*)-4a,5,7a,8,9,9c-Hexahydro-12-methyl-8,9c-imino-
ethanophenanthro[4,5-bcd]furan-3,5-diol monohydrate;
$C_{17}H_{19}NO_3 \cdot H_2O$; relative molecular mass, 303

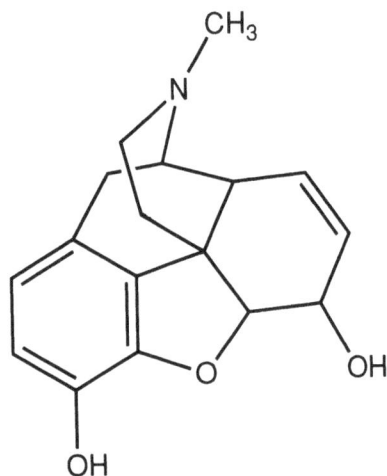

Morphine is the principal alkaloid of opium and is a potent narcotic analgesic. Diamorphine (heroin, 3,6-*O*-diacetylmorphine) has two to three times the potency of morphine and is obtained by treating morphine (or opium in the case of illicit preparations) with acetic anhydride.

Diamorphine is rapidly hydrolysed *in vivo* to 6-acetylmorphine and thence to morphine. Morphine is also a metabolite of codeine. Approximately 5% of a dose of morphine is metabolized to normorphine, but conjugation with glucuronic acid is the major pathway. The principal product is morphine-3-glucuronide, but morphine-6-glucuronide is also formed. Free morphine in urine accounts for about 10% of a dose, while morphine-3-glucuronide accounts for 75%. The estimated minimum fatal dose of morphine or diamorphine in an adult unaccustomed to taking these compounds is 100–200 mg.

Morphine can be detected by thin-layer chromatography of an extract of urine, stomach contents, or scene residues at pH 8.5–9. Since a large proportion of a dose of diamorphine or morphine is excreted as glucuronides, prior hydrolysis of urine can increase the sensitivity of the procedure.

Qualitative test

Applicable to urine.

Reagents

1. Concentrated hydrochloric acid (relative density 1.18).
2. Sodium bicarbonate (solid).
3. Silica gel thin-layer chromatography plate (10 × 20 cm, 20 μm average particle size; see section 4.4.1).
4. Methanol:concentrated ammonium hydroxide (relative density 0.88) (99:1.5) (MA).
5. Ethyl acetate:methanol:concentrated ammonium hydroxide (relative density 0.88) (85:10:5) (EMA).
6. Iodoplatinate reagent. Mix 0.25 g of platinic chloride and 5 g of potassium iodide in 100 ml of purified water.

Standards

1. Hydrolysis standards: codeine, dihydrocodeine and morphine-3-glucuronide (all 1 mg/l) in blank urine.
2. Thin-layer chromatography standards: cocaine, codeine, dihydrocodeine, methadone and morphine (all 1 g/l) in chloroform.

Method

1. Add 2 ml of concentrated hydrochloric acid to 10 ml of urine or hydrolysis standard in a test-tube.
2. Heat on a boiling water-bath for 30 minutes.
3. Allow to cool, decant into a 250 ml beaker and **slowly** add sodium bicarbonate until effervescence ceases and solid sodium bicarbonate remains in the beaker. **Take care — this reaction can be violent.**
4. Decant the hydrolysate into a clean tube, add 10 ml of ethyl acetate:propan-2-ol (9:1) and vortex-mix for 3 minutes.
5. Centrifuge for 5 minutes, filter the upper organic phase through phase-separating filter-paper into a clean tube and discard the lower, aqueous layer.
6. Evaporate the extract to dryness under a stream of compressed air.

Thin-layer chromatography

1. Reconstitute the extracts in 50 μl of ethyl acetate:propan-2-ol (9:1) and spot equal portions of the sample and standard extracts, and 10 μl of the chromatography standard on three columns of two plates.
2. Develop one plate in MA and the second in EMA (10-cm run, saturated tanks, see section 4.4.3).
3. Allow to dry and ensure that no smell of ammonia remains before spraying both plates with iodoplatinate reagent.

Results

The hR$_f$ values and colour reactions of the drugs in the standard mixtures and some additional compounds of interest are given in Table 30. This procedure gives no information as to the presence of diamorphine since this compound and both 3-*O*-acetylmorphine and 6-*O*-acetylmorphine, as well as morphine glucuronides, are hydrolysed to morphine.

The hydrolysis standard extract must be analysed as well as the chromatography standard, since compounds extracted from hydrolysed urine tend to migrate more slowly on thin-layer chromatography owing to the influence of co-extracted compounds, and this must be allowed for in the interpretation of results.

Table 30. Thin-layer chromatography of morphine and related compounds: hR$_f$ values and colour reactions

Compound	hR$_f$		Colour
	EMA	MA	
Methadone metabolite	78	22	Purple
Cocaine[a]	77	73	Violet
Methadone	77	56	Purple (white ring)
Pentazocine	72	71	Speckled blue
Cyclizine	68	68	Speckled dark blue
Dextropropoxyphene metabolite[a]	66	55	Blue (streaks on MA)
Pethidine	62	61	Purple
Nicotine	61	68	Dark brown
Chloroquine	52	44	Dark blue
Quinine	52	70	Speckled blue
6-Acetylmorphine[a]	48	53	Speckled blue
Cotinine (from nicotine)	40	70	Khaki
Hydroxychloroquine	38	53	Blue
Codeine	35	47	Blue
Norpethidine (from pethidine)	34	33	Purple (white rim)
Dihydrocodeine	27	37	Dark blue
Norcotinine (from cotinine)	23	70	Khaki
Desethylchloroquine	22	22	Dark blue
Morphine	20	47	Blue-black
Codeine metabolite	18	25	Blue-purple
Dihydrocodeine metabolite	16	—	Dark blue

[a] Not normally present in urine hydrolysates.

It is important to ensure that only concentrated ammonium hydroxide (relative density 0.88) is used to prepare the mobile phases (MA and EMA) and that a given batch of eluent is used only three times for MA and five times for EMA, as discussed in section 5.2.3.

Sensitivity

Morphine (free + conjugated), 1 mg/l.

Clinical interpretation

Acute poisoning with morphine and diamorphine gives rise to pin-point pupils, hypotension, hypothermia, coma, convulsions and pulmonary oedema. Death may ensue from profound respiratory depression. Naloxone rapidly reverses the central toxic effects of morphine (see section 2.2.2).

6.74 Nicotine

3-(1-Methylpyrrolidin-2-yl)pyridine; $C_{10}H_{14}N_2$; relative molecular mass, 162

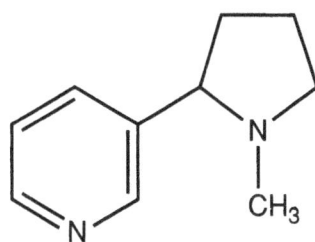

Nicotine is an alkaloid derived from the leaves of *Nicotiana tabacum*. As little as 40 mg of nicotine can prove fatal in an adult. Nicotine is commonly encountered in tobacco although usually in concentrations insufficient to cause acute poisoning, except when ingested by young children. Nicotine occurs in higher concentrations in some herbal medicines, and is also used as a fumigant in horticulture. Nicotine can be absorbed rapidly through the skin, and is metabolized principally by *N*-demethylation to give cotinine.

There is no simple qualitative test for nicotine, but this compound and cotinine can be detected and identified by thin-layer chromatography of a basic solvent extract of urine (see section 5.2.3).

Clinical interpretation

Initially nausea, dizziness, vomiting, respiratory stimulation, headache, tachycardia, sweating and excessive salivation occur followed by collapse, convulsions, cardiac arrhythmias and coma in severe cases. Death may supervene rapidly or be delayed by several hours. Treatment is symptomatic and supportive.

6.75 Nitrates

Nitrates such as sodium nitrate ($NaNO_3$) are most commonly found in inorganic fertilizers, but are also used as antiseptics, food preservatives and explosives. Death in an adult may follow the ingestion of about 15 g of the sodium or potassium salt. Organic nitrates, such as glyceryl trinitrate, are used as vasodilators. Nitrates are metabolized to nitrites in the gastrointestinal tract. Nitrates are strong oxidizing agents and the test given below will also detect compounds with similar properties, such as bromates, chlorates, hypochlorites, iodates and nitrites.

Qualitative test
Applicable to stomach contents and scene residues.

Reagent
Diphenylamine (10 g/l) in concentrated sulfuric acid (relative density 1.83).

Method
1. Filter, if necessary, 5 ml of stomach contents into a 10-ml glass tube.
2. Add 0.5 ml of filtrate or scene residue to a clean tube and **slowly** add 0.5 ml of diphenylamine solution down the side of the tube so that it forms a layer under the sample.

Results
A true positive is indicated by a strong blue colour which develops immediately at the junction of the two layers. A light blue colour will be given by most samples of stomach contents owing to the presence of organic material. Since all strong oxidizing agents are rapidly reduced in biological samples, the test should be performed as soon as possible after receipt of the sample.

Sensitivity
Nitrate, 10 mg/l.

Confirmatory test
Applicable to urine, stomach contents and scene residues.

Reagents

1. Sulfamic acid reagent. Mix 1 ml of ammonium sulfamate (150 g/l) and 1 ml of aqueous hydrochloric acid (2 mol/l), freshly prepared.
2. Aqueous imipramine hydrochloride solution (20 g/l).
3. Concentrated sulfuric acid (relative density 1.83).

Method

1. Mix 0.1 ml of test solution and 0.1 ml of sulfamic acid reagent.
2. Add 0.1 ml of imipramine solution, and **carefully** add 0.2 ml of concentrated sulfuric acid down the side of the tube so that it forms a layer underneath the test mixture.

Results

An intense blue colour at the junction of the two layers confirms nitrate. Sulfamic acid treatment is used to remove any nitrite present prior to the test.

Sensitivity

Nitrate, 50 mg/l.

Clinical interpretation

Acute poisoning with nitrates can cause nausea, vomiting, diarrhoea, abdominal pain, confusion, coma and convulsions. In addition, nitrates may give rise to headache, flushing, dizziness, hypotension and collapse. Treatment is symptomatic and supportive. Methaemoglobinaemia is often produced and this may be indicated by dark chocolate-coloured blood (see section 3.2.2). Blood methaemoglobin can be measured but is unstable and the use of stored samples is unreliable.

6.76 Nitrites

Nitrites such as sodium nitrite ($NaNO_2$) were formerly used as vasodilators, and are used to prevent rusting, as food preservatives and in explosives. Nitrites may also arise from the metabolism of nitrates. The fatal dose of sodium nitrite is about 10 g, although ingestion of as little as 2 g has caused death in an adult. Nitrites are strong oxidizing agents and the test given below will also detect compounds with similar properties such as bromates, chlorates, hypochlorites, iodates and nitrates.

Qualitative test

Applicable to stomach contents and scene residues.

Reagent

Diphenylamine (10 g/l) in concentrated sulfuric acid (relative density 1.83).

Method

1. Filter, if necessary, 5 ml of stomach contents into a 10-ml glass tube.
2. Add 0.5 ml of filtrate or scene residue to a clean tube and **slowly** add 0.5 ml of diphenylamine solution down the side of the tube so that it forms a layer under the sample.

Results

A true positive is indicated by a strong blue colour which develops immediately at the junction of the two layers. A light blue colour will be given by most samples of stomach contents owing to the presence of organic material. Since all strong oxidizing agents are rapidly reduced in biological samples, the test should be performed as soon as possible after receipt of the sample.

Sensitivity

Nitrite, 10 mg/l.

Confirmatory tests

Applicable to urine, stomach contents and scene residues.

1. **Imipramine/hydrochloric acid test**

Reagents

1. Aqueous imipramine hydrochloride (20 g/l).
2. Concentrated hydrochloric acid (relative density 1.18).

Method

To 0.1 ml of imipramine solution add 0.1 ml of test solution and 0.2 ml of hydrochloric acid.

Results

A blue colour is specific for nitrite.

Sensitivity

Nitrite, 1 mg/l.

2. *Sulfanilic acid/1-aminonaphthalene test*

Reagents

1. Sulfanilic acid (10 g/l) in aqueous acetic acid (300 ml/l).
2. 1-Aminonaphthalene (1 g/l) in aqueous acetic acid (300 ml/l).

Method

1. Add 0.1 ml of test solution to 0.1 ml of sulfanilic acid solution.
2. Mix and add 0.1 ml of 1-aminonaphthalene solution.

Results

A purple/red colour is specific for nitrite. If the test solution is strongly acidic or basic the pH should be adjusted beforehand to about 7 (universal indicator paper) by carefully adding 2 mol/l aqueous hydrochloric acid or sodium hydroxide.

Sensitivity

Nitrite, 0.2 mg/l.

Quantitative assay

Applicable to urine.

Reagents

1. Aqueous sodium acetate solution (164 g/l).
2. Sulfanilic acid (6 g/l) in concentrated hydrochloric acid (relative density 1.18):purified water (1:4).
3. 1-Aminonaphthalene (4.8 g/l) in concentrated hydrochloric acid (relative density 1.18):methanol (1:4).

Standards

Solutions containing nitrite ion at concentrations of 0, 10, 20, 50 and 100 mg/l in purified water, prepared by dilution from aqueous sodium nitrite solution (1.50 g/l, equivalent to a nitrite ion concentration of 1.00 g/l).

Method

1. Mix 0.5 ml of sample or standard and 0.5 ml of sulfanilic acid solution in a 25-ml volumetric flask.
2. Allow to stand for 10 minutes, add 0.5 ml of 1-aminonaphthalene solution and 0.5 ml of sodium acetate solution and dilute to 25 ml with purified water.
3. Allow to stand for 10 minutes and measure the absorbance at 510 nm against a water blank carried through the procedure (see section 4.5.2).

Results

Construct a graph of absorbance against nitrite concentration by analysis of the standard solutions and calculate the nitrite concentration in the sample.

Sensitivity

Nitrite, 5 mg/l.

Clinical interpretation

Acute poisoning with nitrites may cause nausea, vomiting, diarrhoea, abdominal pain, confusion, coma and convulsions. In addition, nitrites may give rise to headache, flushing, dizziness, hypotension and collapse. Methaemoglobinaemia is often produced and this may be indicated by dark chocolate-coloured blood (see section 3.2.2). Blood methaemoglobin can be measured but is unstable and the use of stored samples is unreliable. Treatment is symptomatic and supportive. Urinary nitrite ion concentrations of 10 mg/l and above have been reported in fatalities.

6.77 Nitrobenzene

Nitrobenzene (nitrobenzol; $C_6H_5NO_2$; relative molecular mass, 123) has a characteristic odour of bitter almonds and is used in the manufacture of aniline, as a solvent for cellulose ethers, in metal and shoe polishes, perfumes, dyes and soaps, and as a synthetic intermediate. The acute toxicity of nitrobenzene is very similar to that of aniline, probably because of metabolic conversion. Nitrobenzene is metabolized to *p*-aminophenol and *N*-acetyl-*p*-aminophenol (paracetamol), which are both excreted in urine as sulfate and glucuronide conjugates. On hydrolysis of urine, *p*-aminophenol is reformed and can be detected using the *o*-cresol/ammonia test.

Qualitative test

Applicable to urine. *o*-Cresol/ammonia test — see paracetamol monograph (section 6.83).

Results

A strong, royal blue colour developing immediately indicates the presence of *p*-aminophenol. Metabolites of paracetamol (and of phenacetin) also give *p*-aminophenol on hydrolysis and thus interfere. Ethylenediamine (from aminophylline, for example — see section 6.105) gives a green colour in this test.

Sensitivity

p-Aminophenol, 1 mg/l.

Clinical interpretation

Poisoning with nitrobenzene may arise from inhalation or dermal absorption as well as ingestion. Symptoms occur within 1–3 hours of exposure and include confusion, nausea, vomiting and diarrhoea, with convulsions, coma and hepatorenal damage in severe cases. Haemolysis, red (wine-coloured) urine, and methaemoglobinaemia (dark chocolate-coloured blood) are characteristic features of poisoning with nitrobenzene, as with aniline (see section 3.2.2).

Blood methaemoglobin can be measured, but is unstable and the use of stored samples is unreliable. However, hepatic and renal function tests are essential. Treatment may include intravenous methylene blue, but this is contraindicated in patients with glucose-6-phosphate dehydrogenase deficiency, since there is a high risk of inducing haemolysis.

6.78 Nortriptyline

3-(10,11-Dihydro-5H-dibenzo[a,d]cyclohepten-5-ylidene)-N-methyl-propylamine; $C_{19}H_{21}N$; relative molecular mass, 263

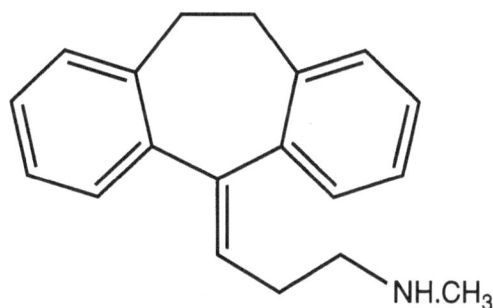

Nortriptyline is the N-demethylated metabolite of amitriptyline and is also a tricyclic antidepressant in its own right.

There is no simple test for nortriptyline, but this compound and other tricyclic antidepressants can be easily detected and identified by thin-layer chromatography of a basic solvent extract of urine, stomach contents or scene residues (see section 5.2.3).

Clinical interpretation

Acute poisoning with nortriptyline and other tricyclic antidepressants may be associated with dilated pupils, hypotension, hypothermia, cardiac arrhythmias, depressed respiration, coma, convulsions and cardiorespiratory arrest. Urinary retention is also a feature of poisoning with these compounds and this may delay procurement of an appropriate specimen for analysis.

Treatment is generally symptomatic and supportive. The use of antiarrhythmic agents is generally avoided, but alkalinization using sodium bicarbonate is sometimes employed. Quantitative measurements in blood are not normally required for management.

6.79 Organochlorine pesticides

These compounds are chlorinated hydrocarbons of diverse structure. Some that may be encountered are listed in Table 31. In addition, benzene hexachloride (BHC) is a mixture of several hexachlorocyclohexane isomers.

These compounds are commonly used as insecticides in many countries, and persist in the environment. Aldrin, dieldrin and endrin (approximate acute lethal dose, 5 g in an adult) are more toxic than lindane or DDT (approximate lethal dose, 30 g).

There are no reliable simple tests for these compounds, although a qualitative analysis can be performed by thin-layer chromatography of a solvent extract of the specimen.

Table 31. Some organochlorine pesticides

Compound	Chemical name	Relative molecular mass
Aldrin (HHDN)	1,2,3,4,10,10-Hexachloro-1,4,4a,5,8,8a-hexahydro-1,4:5,8-dimethanonaphthalene	365
Chlordane	1,2,4,5,6,7,8,8-Octachloro-2,3,3a,4,7,7a-hexahydro-4,7-methanoindene	410
DDT	Principally 1,1,1-trichloro-2,2-bis(4-chloro-phenyl)ethane	355
Dieldrin (HEOD)	1,2,3,4,10,10-Hexachloro-6,7-epoxy-1,4,4a,5,6,7,8,8a-octahydro-*exo*-1,4-*endo*-5,8-dimethanonaphthalene	381
Endrin	1,2,3,4,10,10-Hexachloro-6,7-epoxy-1,4,4a,5,6,7,8,8a-octahydro-*endo*-1,4-*endo*-5,8-dimethanonaphthalene	381
Heptachlor	1,4,5,6,7,8,8-Heptachloro-3a,4,7,7a-tetrahydro-4,7-methanoindene	373
Lindane (γ-HCH)	1α,2α,3β,4α,5α,6β-Hexachlorocyclohexane	291

Qualitative test

Applicable to stomach contents and scene residues.

Reagents

1. Petroleum ether (40-60 °C boiling fraction).
2. Aqueous sodium hydroxide solution (20 g/l).
3. Sodium sulfate (anhydrous).
4. Aqueous potassium permanganate (0.1 mol/l).
5. 2-Aminoethanol (ethanolamine).
6. Silver nitrate reagent. Aqueous silver nitrate (0.1 mol/l):concentrated nitric acid (relative density 1.42) (10:1).
7. Silica gel thin-layer chromatography plate (5 × 20 cm, 20 μm average particle size; see section 4.4.1).

Standards

Aldrin, lindane, dicophane and heptachlor (all 1 g/l) in methanol.

Method

1. Extract 10 ml of sample with 5 ml of petroleum ether for 5 minutes using a rotary mixer.
2. Allow to stand for 5 minutes, take off the upper, ether layer and re-extract with a second 5-ml portion of petroleum ether.
3. Combine the ether extracts and wash with 5-ml portions of:
   (a) purified water;
   (b) sodium hydroxide solution;
   (c) purified water.
4. Filter the extract through phase-separating filter-paper into a clean tube, dry over about 5 g of sodium sulfate and evaporate to dryness under a stream of compressed air or nitrogen.

Thin-layer chromatography

1. Reconstitute the extract in 100 μl of methanol and spot 20 μl on to a column on the plate.
2. Spot 10 μl of the standard mixture on a second column.
3. Develop the chromatogram (10-cm run) using cyclohexane (saturated tank; see section 4.4.3) and allow to dry.
4. Spray the plate with potassium permanganate solution, spray lightly with 2-aminoethanol and heat (preferably in an oven) at 100 °C for 20 minutes.
5. Allow to cool, spray with silver nitrate reagent and expose to ultraviolet light (254 nm) for 15 minutes.

Results

The compounds of interest give brown/black spots. Identification is by comparison with the standard chromatogram. Dieldrin and endrin are not detected under the conditions used. Approximate hR_f values for the remaining compounds are as follows:

lindane 09
dicophane 26
heptachlor 34
aldrin 41

Sensitivity

Organochlorine pesticide, 2.5 mg/l (aldrin 10 mg/l).

Clinical interpretation

Features of poisoning with organochlorine pesticides include vomiting, weakness and numbness of the extremities, apprehension, excitement, diarrhoea and muscular tremor, with convulsions and respiratory depression in severe cases. Treatment is symptomatic and supportive.

6.80 Organophosphorus pesticides

This is a very large group of compounds. There are four basic structures:

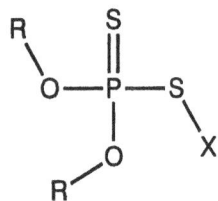

Phosphorodithioates   **Phosphorothioates**

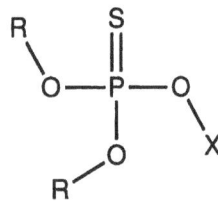

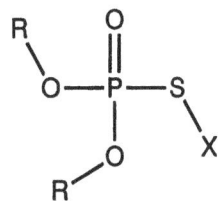

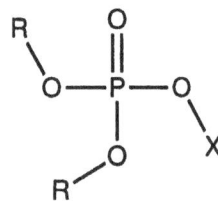

Phosphorothiolates   **Phosphates**

where R = alkyl; X = a wide variety of structures.

An example from each group is given in Table 32. Some organophosphorus pesticides are used as herbicides and are relatively nontoxic to humans. However, most are insecticides which interfere with neurotransmission by inhibition of acetylcholinesterase. This property forms the basis of the confirmatory test described below. Organophosphorus pesticides often have a pungent smell (of garlic), and this property can be helpful in indicating the diagnosis.

Many of these compounds are hydrolysed in alkaline solution while some (for example azinphos-methyl, diazinon, and malathion) are also unstable in acid. For this reason it is important to adjust the pH of stomach contents and scene residues to about 7 prior to the analysis.

Table 32. Some organophosphorus pesticides

Compound	Chemical name	Relative molecular mass
Malathion	Diethyl-2-(dimethoxyphosphinothioylthio) succinate	330
Parathion	*O,O*-Diethyl-*O*-4-nitrophenylphosphorothioate	291
Omethoate	*O,O*-Dimethyl-*S*-methylcarbamoylmethylphosphorothioate	213
Mevinphos	2-Methoxycarbonyl-1-methylvinyldimethyl phosphate	224

Qualitative test

Applicable to stomach contents and scene residues.

Reagents

1. Sodium bicarbonate (solid).
2. Cyclohexane:acetone:chloroform (70:25:5).
3. Acetone:tetraethylenepentamine (9:1).
4. 4-(*p*-Nitrobenzyl)pyridine (20 g/l) in acetone:tetraethylenepentamine (9:1).
5. Silica gel thin-layer chromatography plate (5 × 20 cm, 20 μm average particle size; see section 4.4.1).

Standards

Dimethoate, methidathion, dioxathion and chlorpyrifos (all 1 g/l) in methanol.

Method

1. If necessary, carefully adjust the pH of 10 ml of sample to about 7 by adding solid sodium bicarbonate.
2. Extract 10 ml of sample with 5 ml of methyl tertiary-butyl ether for 5 minutes using a rotary mixer.
3. Allow to stand for 5 minutes, take off the upper, ether layer and re-extract with a second 5-ml portion of methyl tertiary-butyl ether.
4. Combine the extracts, filter through phase-separating filter-paper into a clean tube and evaporate to dryness under a stream of compressed air or nitrogen.

Thin-layer chromatography

1. Reconstitute the extract in 100 μl of methanol and spot 20 μl on a column marked on the plate.
2. Spot 10 μl of the standard mixture on a second column.
3. Develop the chromatogram (10-cm run) using cyclohexane: acetone:chloroform (saturated tank, see section 4.4.3) and allow to dry.
4. Spray the plate with 4-(*p*-nitrobenzyl)pyridine solution and heat, preferably in an oven, at 110 °C for 30 minutes.
5. Allow to cool and spray with acetone:tetraethylenepentamine (9:1).

Results

The compounds of interest give purple spots on a pale brown background. Approximate hR$_f$ values are as follows:

dimethoate	11
methidathion	40
malathion	42
dioxathion	47
propetamphos	49
bromophos	54
chlorpyrifos	58

Sensitivity

Organophosphorus pesticide, 5 mg/l.

Confirmatory test

Applicable to plasma or serum. See cholinesterase activity monograph (section 6.30).

Results

The presence of an acetylcholinesterase inhibitor is indicated if the yellow colour in the control tube is deeper than that in the test tube. If the colour in the tube containing pralidoxime is similar to that in the control tube, this provides further confirmation that an inhibitor of acetylcholinesterase is present in the sample. Of course, other inhibitors of acetylcholinesterase, such as many carbamate pesticides, also give a positive result in this test.

Clinical interpretation

Exposure to organophosphorus insecticides may cause bronchorrhoea, respiratory distress, excessive salivation, nausea, muscle weakness and eventually paralysis. Measurement of erythrocyte cholinesterase activity (see section 3.1.5) provides a method of assessing the severity of poisoning with this group of compounds. Treatment is symptomatic and supportive, and may include the administration of atropine and pralidoxime (see Table 4).

6.81 Orphenadrine

N,N-Dimethyl-2-(2-methylbenzylhydryloxy)ethylamine; $C_{18}H_{23}NO$; relative molecular mass, 269.

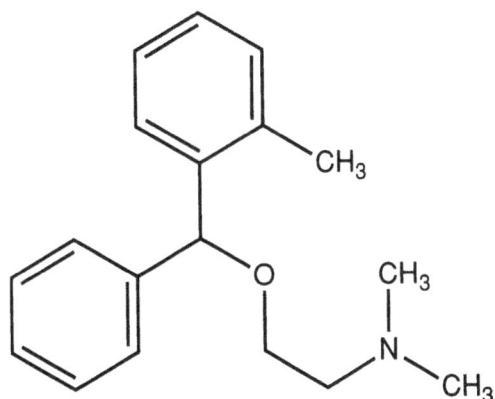

Orphenadrine is an anticholinergic agent used in the treatment of parkinsonism. Up to 60% of an oral dose is excreted in urine within three days. Metabolism is by *N*-demethylation to give *N*-desmethylorphenadrine and *N,N*-didesmethylorphenadrine, *N*-oxidation to give orphenadrine *N*-oxide, and a number of other pathways. The fatal dose of orphenadrine in an adult is thought to be 2–4 g.

There is no simple qualitative test for orphenadrine, but it can be detected and identified by thin-layer chromatography of a basic solvent extract of urine, stomach contents or scene residues (see section 5.2.3).

Clinical interpretation

Acute orphenadrine poisoning may cause a dry mouth, nausea, vomiting, tachycardia, hyperthermia, dizziness, excitement, confusion, hallucinations and convulsions. Treatment is symptomatic and supportive.

6.82 Oxalates

Oxalates are used in bleaching and cleaning agents, metal polishes and anti-rust agents. Oxalic acid ($(COOH)_2 \cdot 2H_2O$; relative molecular mass, 126) also occurs in several plants, the leaves of domestic rhubarb and other members of the dock family (Polygonaceae) containing a particularly high concentration. The fatal dose of oxalic acid in an adult is of the order of 10 g. Oxalic acid is also a major toxic metabolite of ethylene glycol.

Qualitative test

Applicable to urine, stomach contents and scene residues.

Reagents

1. Aqueous calcium chloride solution (100 g/l).
2. Aqueous acetic acid (300 ml/l).
3. Aqueous hydrochloric acid (2 mol/l).

Method

1. Mix 1 ml of calcium chloride solution and 2 ml of clear test solution.
2. If a precipitate forms, add 1 ml of acetic acid.
3. If the precipitate remains, isolate by centrifugation and add 1 ml of dilute hydrochloric acid.

Results

A white precipitate, insoluble in acetic acid, indicates oxalate, fluoride or sulfate. If the precipitate, once isolated, is soluble in dilute hydrochloric acid (step 3), oxalate is indicated.

Sensitivity

Oxalate, 250 mg/l.

Confirmatory tests

1. *Applicable to the precipitate from the qualitative test above.*

Reagents

1. Urea (solid).
2. Thiobarbituric acid (solid) (**not** thiopental — see section 6.9).

Method

1. Wash the precipitate twice with purified water, wash with acetone and dry at room temperature.
2. Suspend the precipitate in 50 μl of methanol in a micro-test-tube and add about 20 mg of urea and about 200 mg of thiobarbituric acid.
3. Mix thoroughly and heat gently on a micro-burner to 140–160 °C.

Results

The rapid formation of a bright orange-red product, soluble in methanol, confirms oxalate.

Sensitivity

Oxalate, 250 mg/l.

2. *Applicable to stomach contents and scene residues.*

Reagents

1. Concentrated ammonium hydroxide (relative density 0.88).
2. Thiobarbituric acid (solid) (**not** thiopental — see section 6.9).

Method

1. Mix 50 μl of test solution with 100 μl of concentrated ammonium hydroxide in a micro-test-tube and carefully evaporate to dryness using a micro-burner.
2. Add about 200 mg of thiobarbituric acid and gently reheat to 140–160 °C.

Results

The rapid formation of a bright orange-red product, soluble in methanol, confirms oxalate.

Sensitivity

Oxalate, 250 mg/l.

Clinical interpretation

In addition to irritant effects on the alimentary tract when ingested, oxalate sequesters calcium, causing hypocalcaemia, muscular twitching and eventually tetany, convulsions, flank pain, acute renal failure and cardiac arrest. The crystalluria produced may be diagnostic (section 5.2.1). Treatment is normally symptomatic and supportive.

6.83 Paracetamol

Acetaminophen; *N*-acetyl-*p*-aminophenol; $C_8H_9NO_2$; relative molecular mass, 151

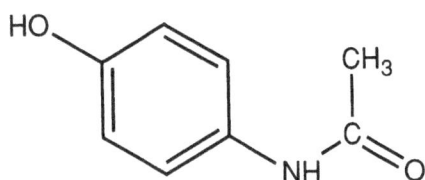

Paracetamol is a widely used analgesic and sometimes occurs in combination with other drugs such as dextropropoxyphene. It is a metabolite of phenacetin and of benorilate, and is itself largely metabolized by conjugation with glucuronic acid and sulfate prior to urinary excretion.

Hydrolysis of the glucuronate and sulfate conjugates with concentrated hydrochloric acid gives *p*-aminophenol, which can be conjugated with *o*-cresol to form a strongly coloured dye, thus giving a sensitive qualitative test. Protein precipitation with trichloroacetic acid and subsequent treatment with nitrous acid and spectrophotometric measurement of the nitrated derivative give a selective assay for paracetamol in plasma.

Qualitative test
Applicable to urine, stomach contents and scene residues.

Reagents
1. Concentrated hydrochloric acid (relative density 1.18).
2. Aqueous *o*-cresol solution (10 g/l).
3. Aqueous ammonium hydroxide solution (4 mol/l).

Method
1. Add 0.5 ml of hydrochloric acid to 0.5 ml of sample, boil for 10 minutes and cool.
2. Add 1 ml of *o*-cresol solution to 0.2 ml of the hydrolysate.
3. Add 2 ml of ammonium hydroxide solution and mix for 5 seconds.

Results

A strong, royal blue colour developing immediately indicates the presence of paracetamol. This test is very sensitive and will detect therapeutic dosage with paracetamol 24–48 hours later.

Only aromatic amines, such as aniline, which also give rise to *p*-aminophenol in urine after hydrolysis are known to interfere. Ethylene-diamine (from aminophylline, for example; see section 6.105) gives a green colour in this test.

Sensitivity

p-Aminophenol, 1 mg/l.

Quantitative assay

Applicable to plasma or serum.

Reagents

1. Aqueous trichloroacetic acid (100 g/l).
2. Aqueous hydrochloric acid (6 mol/l).
3. Aqueous sodium nitrite solution (100 g/l, freshly prepared).
4. Aqueous ammonium sulfamate solution (150 g/l).
5. Aqueous sodium hydroxide solution (6 mol/l).

Standards

Prepare solutions containing paracetamol at concentrations of 0, 50, 100, 200 and 400 mg/l in blank plasma. These solutions are unstable even at 4 °C and must be prepared weekly or stored at − 20 °C.

Method

1. Add 2 ml of trichloroacetic acid to 1 ml of sample or standard, mix and centrifuge for 5 minutes
2. In a separate tube add 1 ml of hydrochloric acid to 2 ml of sodium nitrite solution and mix. **Take care — brown nitrogen dioxide fumes may be evolved**.
3. Add 2.0 ml of the supernatant from step 1 to the mixture obtained in step 2, mix, and allow to stand for 2–3 minutes at room temperature.
4. Add 2 ml of ammonium sulfamate solution drop by drop to remove excess nitrous acid. **Take care** — vigorous frothing occurs.
5. Add 2 ml of sodium hydroxide solution, vortex-mix to remove any gas bubbles and measure the absorbance at 450 nm against a plasma blank (see section 4.5.2).

Results

Calculate the plasma paracetamol concentration by comparison with the results obtained from the standard solutions. Paracetamol metabolites do not interfere, but the method is only useful within 4–24 hours of ingestion and the limit of sensitivity (normally 50 mg/l) may be 100 mg/l or more with uraemic sera.

Salicylic acid interferes to a small extent: a salicylate concentration of 1 g/l gives an apparent paracetamol concentration of 50 mg/l. However, 4-aminosalicylic acid reacts strongly (100 mg/l gives an apparent paracetamol concentration of 320 mg/l). Levodopa also interferes, and specimens contaminated with mucous heparin or other solutions containing *o*-cresol preservative can give very high false readings.

Sensitivity

Paracetamol, 50 mg/l.

Clinical interpretation

Following paracetamol overdosage only mild symptoms, such as nausea and vomiting, may occur initially, but severe, possibly fatal, hepatic damage may develop within days of the ingestion. Renal damage also occurs in a proportion of patients. Treatment with methionine or acetylcysteine (*N*-acetylcysteine) can protect against such damage if given within 12–15 hours of the overdose (see Table 6, p. 11).

Fig. 12. Interpretation of plasma paracetamol results

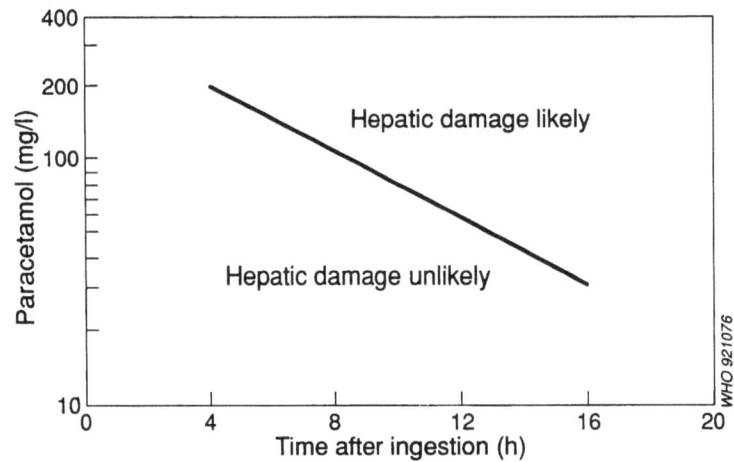

Treatment with methionine or acetylcysteine is indicated if the plasma concentration is above the line. Results obtained within 4 hours of ingestion are unreliable and should be used with caution, since absorption may not be complete.

Since indicators of hepatic damage such as prothrombin time (see section 3.2.1) may only become abnormal at 12–36 hours, measurement of the plasma paracetamol concentration is important not only in establishing the diagnosis, but also in assessing the need for protective therapy (Fig. 12). However, the qualitative urine test given above should be performed if there is any suspicion that paracetamol has been ingested, especially in patients presenting 24 hours or more after ingestion.

6.84 Paraquat

1,1'-Dimethyl-4,4'-bipyridylium ion; $C_{12}H_{14}N_2$; relative molecular mass, 186

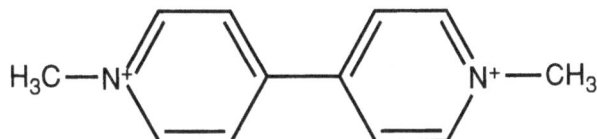

Paraquat is a widely used contact herbicide and may be formulated together with the related herbicide diquat. Paraquat is often encountered as the dichloride and is extremely poisonous — the lethal dose in an adult may be as low as 4 mg/kg of body weight. Paraquat and diquat give highly coloured products with sodium dithionite, and this reaction forms the basis of the test described.

Qualitative test
Applicable to urine, stomach contents and scene residues.

Reagents
1. Sodium dithionite (solid, stored in a desiccator).
2. Aqueous ammonium hydroxide (2 mol/l).
3. Blank urine.
4. Urine specimen containing paraquat ion (10 mg/l). **Take care — paraquat is very toxic and may be absorbed through the skin.**

Method
1. Add 0.5 ml of ammonium hydroxide solution to 1 ml of test solution, and to 1-ml portions of blank and standard urines in separate test-tubes.
2. Add about 20 mg of sodium dithionite to each tube and mix.
3. If any colour forms in the test solution, agitate in air for several minutes.

Results

A blue/blue-black colour indicates the presence of paraquat. The related herbicide diquat gives a yellow-green colour, but interference from this compound is insignificant in the presence of paraquat.

If the colour fades on continued agitation in air, paraquat/diquat is confirmed — the original colour can be restored by adding more sodium dithionite.

Sensitivity

Paraquat, 1 mg/l.

Clinical interpretation

Ingestion of paraquat may cause a burning sensation in the mouth, oesophagus and abdomen together with ulceration of the lips, tongue and pharynx. After massive absorption of paraquat, the patient usually dies quickly from multiple organ failure. Absorption of lower doses may lead to the development of progressive pulmonary fibrosis, which ultimately causes death from respiratory failure. Myocardial and renal failure may also occur. Treatment is symptomatic and supportive. Measures to reduce absorption (by the oral administration of Fuller's earth or activated charcoal) or enhance elimination (by haemodialysis) of paraquat have not been shown to affect the outcome.

The major role of an analysis is to assess the prognosis in patients at risk from progressive pulmonary fibrosis; a strongly positive result in a urine sample obtained more than 4 hours after ingestion indicates a poor prognosis. Plasma paraquat concentrations can be measured as a prognostic guide, but reliable methods require either radioimmunoassay or high-performance liquid chromatography.

6.85 Pentachlorophenol

PCP; C_6HCl_5O; relative molecular mass, 266

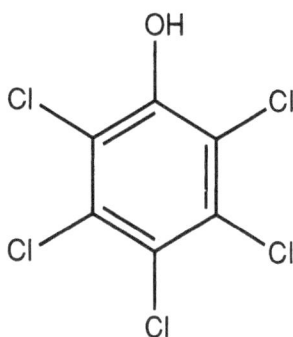

Pentachlorophenol is widely used in wood preservatives and disinfectants, and as a contact herbicide. Pentachlorophenol uncouples oxidative phosphorylation, and poisoning can occur as a result of occupational exposure as well as ingestion. Unlike the dinitrophenol pesticides, there is no yellow staining of the skin, but pentachlorophenol has a characteristic phenolic smell and this may help the diagnosis.

Qualitative test

Applicable to stomach contents and scene residues.

Reagents

1. Aqueous sodium hydroxide solution (2 mol/l).
2. Concentrated sulfuric acid (relative density 1.83).
3. Concentrated nitric acid (relative density 1.40).

Method

1. Mix 10 ml of sample and 20 ml of *n*-butyl acetate for 5 minutes using a rotary mixer and centrifuge for 5 minutes.
2. Transfer the extract to a clean tube and evaporate to dryness on a boiling water-bath under a stream of compressed air or nitrogen.
3. Add 0.2 ml of concentrated nitric acid to the residue and heat the tube in the boiling water-bath for 30 seconds.
4. Cool and add 0.1 ml of the mixture to 2 ml of concentrated sulfuric acid.
5. To the remainder of the cooled mixture add 2 ml of purified water and then add sodium hydroxide solution drop by drop until the pH reaches 8 (universal indicator paper).

Results

Pentachlorophenol gives a red colour in steps 3 and 4 and a brown-violet colour in step 5. Other chlorinated phenols such as hexachlorophane also react in this test.

Sensitivity

Pentachlorophenol, 1 g/l.

Clinical interpretation

Exposure to pentachlorophenol may cause sweating, hyperpyrexia, increased respiratory rate and tachycardia. Death has occurred in severe cases. Since acute poisoning occurs commonly by skin and pulmonary absorption, the prevention of further absorption is important as well as symptomatic and supportive measures.

6.86 Peroxides

Hydrogen peroxide (H_2O_2) is an oxidizing agent used as a bleach and sterilizing agent in cosmetics and other household products, and in industry. It is often encountered as a relatively dilute aqueous solution (60 ml/l or "20 volume", meaning that 1 volume of liquid can release 20 volumes of oxygen), but concentrations of up to 300 ml/l ("100 volume") are used in industry.

Solid metallic peroxides such as barium peroxide (BaO_2) and magnesium peroxide (MgO_2) are very strong oxidizing agents. These compounds have various industrial uses and liberate hydrogen peroxide on treatment with dilute acid. Some organic peroxides are used as catalysts in the production of epoxy resins.

Qualitative test

Applicable to stomach contents and scene residues.

Reagents

1. Aqueous hydrochloric acid (2 mol/l).
2. Aqueous potassium dichromate solution (100 g/l).
3. Aqueous sulfuric acid (2 mol/l).

Method

1. If the suspect material is a solid, carefully prepare a paste (about 1 g) with water and add to 10 ml of cold dilute hydrochloric acid.
2. Add 1 ml of liquid test solution (or 1 ml of the acidified solution prepared above) to 1 ml of potassium dichromate solution, 1 ml of dilute sulfuric acid and 2 ml of diethyl ether.
3. Vortex-mix for 30 seconds and allow the phases to separate.

Results

A blue colour in the ether layer indicates the presence of hydrogen peroxide, either in the test solution or by liberation from a metal peroxide.

Sensitivity

Hydrogen peroxide, 100 mg/l.

Confirmatory test

Applicable to stomach contents and scene residues.

Reagents

1. Aqueous lead acetate solution (100 g/l).

2. Hydrogen sulfide gas (cylinder). **Avoid inhalation of hydrogen sulfide—it has a strong smell of rotten eggs at low concentration and is very toxic.**

Method

1. Soak a strip of filter-paper in the lead acetate solution, expose to hydrogen sulfide **in a fume cupboard**, and allow to dry.
2. Spot 0.1 ml of liquid test solution or 0.1 ml of the acidified solution prepared for the qualitative test on the paper.

Results

A white spot is formed on the brown-black paper if hydrogen peroxide is present owing to the oxidation of lead sulfide to sulfate.

Sensitivity

Hydrogen peroxide, 500 mg/l.

Clinical interpretation

Ingestion of hydrogen peroxide gives rise to a burning sensation in the mouth, throat and oesophagus. However, there are usually no primary systemic effects, since decomposition to water and oxygen occurs before absorption. Poisoning with metallic peroxides is very rare, but these compounds are powerful oxidizing and corrosive agents and can give rise to systemic toxicity attributable to the metallic component. Treatment is symptomatic and supportive.

6.87 Pethidine

Meperidine; ethyl 1-methyl-4-phenylpiperidine-4-carboxylate; $C_{15}H_{21}NO_2$; relative molecular mass, 247

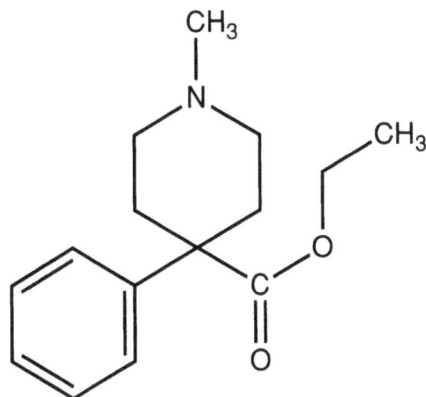

Pethidine is a narcotic analgesic. About 45% of an oral dose is metabolized by N-demethylation to norpethidine, by hydrolysis to pethidinic acid, and by a number of other pathways. Up to approximately 30% of a dose is excreted in urine as pethidine and norpethidine under acidic conditions, but only 5% is excreted as these compounds if the urine is alkaline.

There is no simple qualitative test for pethidine, but this compound and its metabolites can be detected and identified by thin-layer chromatography of a basic solvent extract of urine (see section 5.2.3).

Clinical interpretation

Acute overdosage with pethidine may give rise to pin-point pupils, hypotension, hypothermia, coma and convulsions. Death may ensue from profound respiratory depression, but fatalities are relatively rare. Naloxone rapidly reverses the central toxic effects of pethidine (see section 2.2.2).

6.88 Petroleum distillates

Petrol (gasoline) is largely a mixture of normal and branched-chain aliphatic hydrocarbons (C_4–C_{12}) with boiling points in the range 39–204 °C. Paraffin (kerosene) is a higher boiling fraction. Acute poisoning with petrol usually arises from inhalation of vapour as a result of industrial accident or deliberate abuse (sniffing or ingestion). Tetraethyl lead is frequently added to petrol to prevent pre-ignition (anti-knock) and chronic organo-lead poisoning can follow long-term abuse.

There are no simple qualitative tests for petroleum distillates. However, the characteristic smell of petrol on the breath or from stomach contents (or even postmortem tissue) may help to indicate the diagnosis.

Clinical interpretation

Headache, dizziness, nausea, vomiting, confusion, tremor, disorientation, coma and cardiac arrhythmias may occur after oral ingestion of petrol or sublethal inhalation of petrol vapour. The aspiration of even small quantities of petrol may lead to chemical pneumonitis. The inhalation of high concentrations of vapour may be rapidly fatal, with acute respiratory failure or cardiorespiratory arrest.

6.89 Phenacetin

p-Ethoxyacetanilide; acetophenetidin; $C_{10}H_{13}NO_2$; relative molecular mass, 179

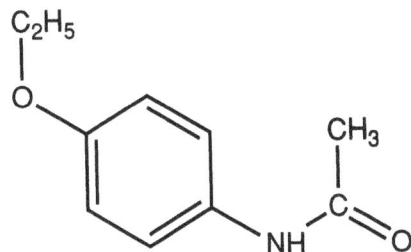

Phenacetin was previously used as an analgesic, but long-term use was associated with nephrotoxicity. It is largely metabolized to paracetamol and thus ingestion of phenacetin can be detected in urine using the *o*-cresol/ammonia test on a hydrolysed urine specimen.

Qualitative test

Applicable to urine. *o*-Cresol/ammonia test—see paracetamol monograph (section 6.83).

Results

A strong, royal blue colour developing immediately indicates the presence of paracetamol. This test is very sensitive and will detect therapeutic dosage with phenacetin 24–48 hours later.

Only aromatic amines such as aniline, which also give rise to *p*-aminophenol in urine after hydrolysis, are known to interfere. Ethylenediamine (from aminophylline, for example; see section 6.105) gives a green colour in this test.

Sensitivity

p-Aminophenol, 1 mg/l.

Clinical interpretation

Acute ingestion of phenacetin can cause dizziness, euphoria, cyanosis, haemolytic anaemia, respiratory depression, and cardiorespiratory arrest. Methaemoglobinaemia is often produced and may be indicated by dark chocolate-coloured blood (see section 3.2.2). Blood methaemoglobin can be measured, but is unstable and the use of stored samples is unreliable. Although metabolized to paracetamol, phenacetin does not cause acute hepatorenal necrosis. Treatment is symptomatic and supportive.

6.90 Phenols

Phenol (hydroxybenzene; carbolic acid; C_6H_5OH; relative molecular mass, 94) and cresol (cresylic acid; $CH_3.C_6H_4OH$; relative molecular mass, 108) are used as disinfectants and in the plastics industry. Commercial cresol is a mixture of *o*-, *m*-, and *p*-cresols in which the *m*-isomer predominates. The estimated minimum lethal dose of phenol or cresol in an adult is 1–2 g.

Both phenol and cresol are readily absorbed through the skin and via the gastrointestinal tract when ingested. They are excreted in urine mainly as glucuronide or sulfate conjugates.

Qualitative test

Applicable to urine.

Reagents

1. Folin-Ciocalteau reagent. Dissolve 100 g of sodium tungstate and 25 g of sodium molybdate in 800 ml of purified water in a 1.5-l flask. Add 50 ml of concentrated orthophosphoric acid (840–900 g/kg) and 100 ml of concentrated hydrochloric acid (relative density 1.18) and reflux for 10 hours. Cool, add 150 g of lithium sulfate, 50 ml of purified water and 0.5 ml of elemental bromine, and allow to stand for 2 hours. Boil for 15 minutes to remove excess bromine, cool, filter if necessary, and dilute to 1 litre with purified water. This solution is yellow and should be stable for 4 months if stored at 4 °C. Folin-Ciocalteau reagent can also be purchased ready-made.
2. Aqueous sodium hydroxide solution (2 mol/l).

Method

1. Dilute 1 ml of Folin-Ciocalteau reagent with 2 ml of purified water and add 1 ml of urine.
2. Add 1 ml of sodium hydroxide solution and vortex-mix for 5 seconds.

Results

A blue colour indicates the presence of a phenolic compound. Halogenated phenols such as 2,4,6-trichlorophenol react less strongly than nonhalogenated phenols.

Sensitivity

Phenol, 10 mg/l.

Clinical interpretation

Phenols burn and cause depigmentation of the skin, and corrode the lips and mouth if ingested. In severe poisoning, nausea, vomiting, abdominal pain, gastric haemorrhage or perforation, metabolic acidosis, coma, hypotension and shock may occur. Death from respiratory depression may ensue. Hepatorenal failure is an additional complication, and the urine may become dark-coloured owing to the presence of free haemoglobin. Apart from skin decontamination with castor oil or olive oil, treatment is symptomatic and supportive.

6.91 Phenothiazines

These compounds are derivatives of phenothiazine, which itself is used as an anthelminthic in veterinary medicine.

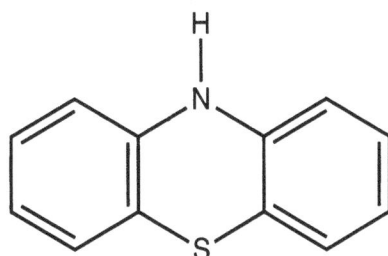

Some commonly encountered phenothiazines are listed in Table 33.

Phenothiazines are widely used as antihistamines, tranquillizers, and in various psychiatric disorders. They are often extensively metabolized. Chloropromazine, for example, has over 50 metabolites in humans. The test described below is based on the reaction of many of these compounds with ferric ion under acidic conditions.

Phenothiazines are often detected during thin-layer chromatography of basic solvent extracts of urine (see section 5.2.3), but specific identification of the compound ingested may be impossible if only urine is available. Low-dose phenothiazines, such as fluphenazine, may not be detectable in urine using either method.

Qualitative test

Applicable to urine, stomach contents and scene residues.

Reagent

FPN reagent. Mix 5 ml of aqueous ferric chloride solution (50 g/l), 45 ml of aqueous perchloric acid (200 g/kg) and 50 ml of aqueous nitric acid (500 ml/l).

Table 33. Some common phenothiazines

Compound	Chemical name	Relative molecular mass
Chlorpromazine	3-(2-Chlorophenothiazin-10-yl)-*N,N*-dimethylpropylamine	319
Chlorprothixene	(Z)-3-(2-Chlorothioxanthen-9-ylidene)-*N,N*-dimethylpropylamine	316
Dimetotiazine	10-(2-Dimethylaminopropyl)-*N,N*-dimethylphenothiazine-2-sulfonamide	392
Prochlorperazine	2-Chloro-10-[3-(4-methylpiperazin-1-yl)propyl]phenothiazine	374
Promazine	*N,N*-Dimethyl-3-(phenothiazin-10-yl)propylamine	284
Promethazine	1,*N,N*-Trimethyl-2-(phenothiazin-10-yl)ethylamine	284
Thioridazine	10-[2-(1-Methyl-2-piperidyl)ethyl]-2-methylthiophenothiazine	371

Method

Add 1 ml of FPN reagent to 1 ml of sample and mix for 5 seconds.

Results

Colours ranging from pink, red or orange to violet or blue may indicate the presence of phenothiazines or metabolites. Urine from patients on chronic treatment with conventional phenothiazines, such as chlorpromazine, will usually give a positive reaction.

Tricyclic antidepressants such as imipramine may also give green or blue colours. False positive reactions may be obtained in patients with phenylketonuria or hepatic impairment.

Sensitivity

Chlorpromazine, 25 mg/l.

Clinical interpretation

Features of acute poisoning with phenothiazines include drowsiness, tremor, restlessness, hyperreflexia, hypothermia, hypotension, hypoventilation, convulsions, tachycardia and cardiac arrhythmias. Phenothiazine overdosage is not normally associated with a fatal outcome, although serious poisoning with, for example, chlorpromazine has been described. Treatment is normally symptomatic and supportive.

6.92 Phenytoin

Diphenylhydantoin; 5,5-diphenylimidazolidine-2,4-dione; $C_{15}H_{12}N_2O_2$; relative molecular mass, 252

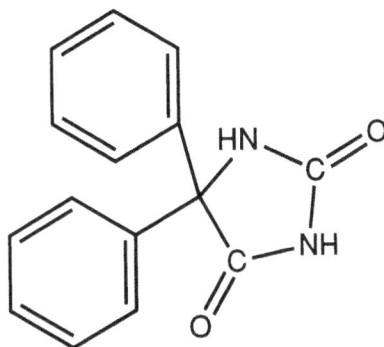

Phenytoin is a widely used anticonvulsant. Metabolic pathways include aromatic hydroxylation and conjugation, less than 5% of a dose being excreted unchanged in urine. The estimated minimum lethal dose in an adult is 5 g, but few fatal overdoses involving this compound alone have been reported.

There is no simple qualitative test for phenytoin, but it can be detected and identified by thin-layer chromatography of an acidic solvent extract of urine, stomach contents or scene residues (see section 5.2.3).

Clinical interpretation

Features of phenytoin poisoning include tremor, nystagmus, ataxia, coma and respiratory depression. Intravenous overdosage may be associated with cardiac toxicity. Treatment is normally symptomatic and supportive. Haemoperfusion may be of value in severe cases.

6.93 Phosphorus and phosphides

Yellow phosphorus (P) and the phosphides of zinc, aluminium and magnesium are used as rodenticides, usually as a paste containing sugar and bran.

Qualitative test

Applicable to stomach contents and scene residues.

Reagents

1. Silver nitrate solution (saturated) in methanol.
2. Aqueous lead acetate solution (100 g/l).

Method

1. Soak a strip (5 × 1 cm) of filter-paper in the silver nitrate solution and allow to dry at room temperature.
2. Soak a similar strip of filter-paper in the lead acetate solution and again dry at room temperature.
3. Place 5 ml of sample in a boiling-tube fitted with a cork with a slit cut in each side.
4. Insert the test papers into the slits, stopper the tube and heat on a water-bath at 60 °C for 20 minutes.

Results

If only the silver nitrate paper is blackened then phosphorus or phosphides may be present. If both papers are blackened then sulfides may be present and the result is inconclusive.

Sensitivity

Phosphorus, 1 g/l.

Confirmatory test

Applicable to blackened silver nitrate paper from the test above.

Reagents

1. Ammonium molybdate reagent. Mix 5 g of ammonium molybdate in 100 ml of water and 35 ml of concentrated nitric acid (relative density 1.42).
2. *o*-Toluidine reagent. Mix 50 mg of *o*-toluidine and 10 ml of glacial acetic acid, diluted to 100 ml with purified water.
3. Concentrated ammonium hydroxide (relative density 0.88).
4. Powdered calcium hypochlorite.

Method

1. Place the silver nitrate paper on a glass microscope slide and cover with calcium hypochlorite.
2. Leave in a moist chamber for 15 minutes to allow oxidation of phosphide to phosphate.
3. Remove excess hypochlorite by careful washing with a small amount of purified water and dry the test paper by blotting with absorbent tissue.
4. Add 50 μl of ammonium molybdate reagent to the dried paper followed by 50 μl of *o*-toluidine reagent and expose the paper to ammonia fumes from concentrated ammonium hydroxide **in a fume cupboard**.

Results

A blue colour confirms phosphorus.

Sensitivity

Phosphorus, 1 g/l.

Clinical interpretation

Acute poisoning with yellow phosphorus gives rise to gastrointestinal corrosion, nausea and vomiting, leading to coma, hypotension and hepatorenal damage. Phosphides release phosphine (PH_3) on contact with water or moist air, and this gas acts on the gastrointestinal and central nervous systems. Abdominal pain may be followed by nausea, vomiting, gross ataxia, convulsions and coma, with death, usually within 2 hours, in severe cases. Treatment is symptomatic and supportive.

6.94 Procainamide

4-Amino-*N*-(2-diethylaminoethyl)benzamide; $C_{13}H_{21}N_3O$; relative molecular mass, 235

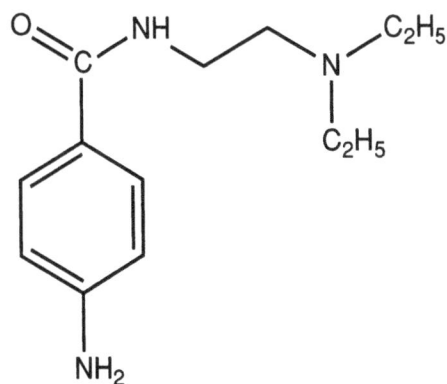

Procainamide is a widely used antiarrhythmic drug. The major metabolite, *N*-acetylprocainamide (NAPA) has similar pharmacological activity to the parent compound. Up to 80% of a dose is excreted in urine in 24 hours, some 50–60% as procainamide and about 30% as NAPA. The normal oral dose is 0.5–1 g of procainamide every 4–6 hours, but as little as 200 mg given intravenously may prove fatal.

There is no simple qualitative test for procainamide, but this compound and NAPA can be detected and identified by thin-layer chromatography of a basic solvent extract of urine (see section 5.2.3).

Clinical interpretation

Acute poisoning with procainamide may cause anorexia, nausea, vomiting, diarrhoea and cardiac arrhythmias. Rapid intravenous injection may cause hypotension, convulsions and collapse. Treatment is symptomatic and supportive.

6.95 Propan-2-ol

iso-Propanol; *iso*-propyl alcohol; $CH_3.CHOH.CH_3$; relative molecular mass, 60

Propan-2-ol is used in lotions for topical administration, in window and screen washers, and as a solvent for toiletries. It is also used as a vehicle for certain pharmaceutical preparations and serious iatrogenic poisoning has occurred in children. The estimated minimum fatal dose of propan-2-ol in an adult is 240 ml.

Propan-2-ol is metabolized to acetone by alcohol dehydrogenase. The qualitative test described below relies on the oxidation of propan-2-ol to acetone and subsequent detection of acetone. Note that propan-2-ol is often used as a topical antiseptic prior to venepuncture, and care must be taken to avoid contamination of the sample if poisoning with this agent is suspected.

Qualitative test
Applicable to plasma or serum.

Reagents
1. Salicylaldehyde solution (100 ml/l) in methanol.
2. Aqueous sodium hydroxide solution (300 g/l).
3. Potassium permanganate reagent. Mix 3 g of potassium permanganate, 15 ml of orthophosphoric acid (850 g/kg) and 85 ml of purified water.
4. Aqueous trichloroacetic acid solution (200 g/l).
5. Sodium bisulfite (solid).

Method
1. Add 1 ml of plasma or serum to 2 ml of trichloroacetic acid solution, vortex-mix for 30 seconds and centrifuge for 5 minutes.
2. Transfer 1 ml of the supernatant to a second tube and add 0.3 ml of potassium permanganate reagent.
3. Vortex-mix for 5 seconds and allow to stand for 10 minutes. If the pink coloration fades continue to add 0.1-ml portions of potassium permanganate reagent until the colour persists.

4. Decolorize by adding solid sodium bisulfite (about 100 mg).

5. Add 3 ml of sodium hydroxide solution and 0.1 ml of salicylaldehyde solution and vortex-mix for 5 seconds.

6. Heat in a boiling water-bath for 4 minutes and cool.

Results

A red colour indicates the presence of propan-2-ol or acetone.

Sensitivity

Propan-2-ol, 50 mg/l.

Clinical interpretation

Initial symptoms of poisoning with propan-2-ol are similar to those of ethanol and include inebriation, nausea, vomiting and abdominal pain. Serious poisoning is rare but features include haemorrhagic gastritis, coma, respiratory depression, hypothermia, renal failure, rhabdomyolysis, myoglobinuria, haemolytic anaemia and ketonuria. Treatment is supportive and may include haemodialysis in severe cases.

The half-life of acetone is much longer than that of propan-2-ol so that the later signs of poisoning observed are largely those of acetone. Acetone can be detected on the breath of patients poisoned with propan-2-ol. A simple dip-strip test for urinary acetone is available.

6.96 Propranolol

($\pm$)-1-Isopropylamino-3-(1-naphthyloxy)propan-2-ol; $C_{16}H_{21}NO_2$; relative molecular mass, 259

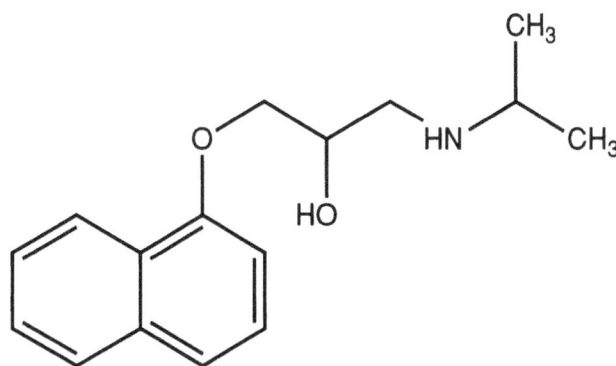

Propranolol is a β-adrenoceptor-blocking agent (β-blocker). It is given orally in the treatment of hypertension and some cardiac disorders, and has a variety of other uses. Propranolol undergoes extensive first-pass metabolism, and metabolic pathways include aromatic hydroxylation, N-dealkylation, oxidative deamination and conjugation.

There is no simple qualitative test for propranolol, but this compound and some of its metabolites may be detected and identified by thin-layer chromatography of a basic solvent extract of urine (see section 5.2.3).

Clinical interpretation

Overdosage with propranolol and other β-blockers may cause delirium, hallucinations, bradycardia, hypotension, bronchospasm, hypoglycaemia, coma and convulsions. Death may follow low-output cardiac failure or cardiorespiratory arrest. Treatment may include the administration of atropine, glucagon and β-agonists.

6.97 Propylene glycol

Propane-1,2-diol; $CH_3.CHOH.CH_2OH$; relative molecular mass, 76

Propylene glycol is widely used as a solvent in the pharmaceutical and food industries, usually as a 100 ml/l or 200 ml/l aqueous solution, and in veterinary practice. It has a relatively short plasma half-life (4–8 hours), and is metabolized primarily to lactic and pyruvic acids, although a large proportion (20–30%) of a dose is excreted unchanged in urine.

Propylene glycol is relatively safe in normal use, but cases of poisoning associated with its use as a vehicle for drugs or vitamins given intravenously or orally have been described. Plasma concentrations associated with serious toxicity are over 4 g/l, corresponding in adults to the administration of 100–200 ml of intravenous fluids containing 200–300 ml/l propylene glycol over a relatively short time.

There is no simple qualitative test for propylene glycol.

Clinical interpretation

Overdosage with propylene glycol may cause lactic acidosis, haemolysis, coma, convulsions and cardiorespiratory arrest. Increased plasma osmolality can be a useful but nonspecific indicator of poisoning with this compound (see section 3.1.3).

6.98 Quinine and quinidine

These compounds have the structure:

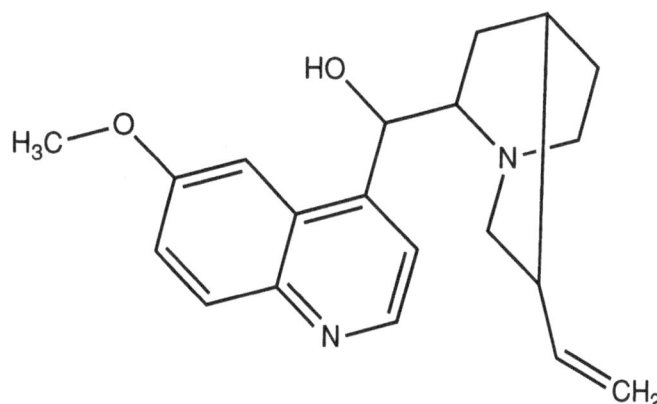

Quinine ((8S,9R)-6'-methoxycinchonan-9-ol trihydrate; $C_{20}H_{24}N_2O_2 \cdot 3H_2O$; relative molecular mass, 379) is the dextrorotatory stereo-isomer of quinidine ((8r,9s)-6'-methoxycinchonan-9-ol dihydrate; $C_{20}H_{24}N_2O_2 \cdot 2H_2O$; relative molecular mass, 361). Commercial samples of either compound may contain up to 10% or 30% of hydroquinine or hydroquinidine, respectively.

Quinine is the major alkaloid found in the bark of various species of *Cinchona* and is used in the treatment of malaria. It is also used to treat night cramps and is a constituent of tonic water. The fatal dose of quinine in an adult may be as little as 8 g. Quinidine is used as an antiarrhythmic. Both compounds are extensively metabolized, largely to hydroxylated metabolites.

Qualitative test

Applicable to urine.

Reagents

1. Aqueous hydrochloric acid (2 mol/l).
2. Sodium chloride (solid).

Method

1. Add 0.1 ml of dilute hydrochloric acid to 1 ml of sample and vortex-mix for 10 seconds.
2. Examine under ultraviolet light (366 nm).
3. If fluorescence is observed, add about 1 g of sodium chloride and vortex-mix for 30 seconds.

Results

If any fluorescence observed at step 2 is due to quinine/quinidine then it will be largely, if not completely, quenched by addition of sodium chloride.

In addition to the above, quinine and quinidine and their metabolites can be detected and identified by thin-layer chromatography of a basic solvent extract of urine (see section 5.2.3). However, care may be needed to differentiate these compounds from emetine if syrup of ipecacuanha has been used to induce vomiting (see section 2.2.1 and Table 15).

Sensitivity

Quinine or quinidine, 50 mg/l.

Clinical interpretation

Overdosage with quinine may cause nausea, vomiting, abdominal pain, diarrhoea, tinnitus, deafness, vertigo, headache, blurred vision, blindness (which may be permanent), hypotension, coma, acute renal failure and cardiorespiratory arrest. In addition to general supportive measures, repeat-dose oral activated charcoal may be used to enhance systemic elimination of quinine. The efficacy of stellate ganglion block in preventing retinal damage has not been established.

The gastrointestinal and cerebellar signs of acute quinidine poisoning are similar to those caused by quinine. However, metabolic and circulatory effects predominate, and include hypotension, hypokalaemia, hypocalcaemia, hypophosphataemia, hypomagnesaemia, metabolic acidosis, acute renal failure, coma, convulsions, cardiac arrhythmias and circulatory collapse. Treatment is largely symptomatic and supportive.

6.99 Salicylic acid and derivatives

Salicylic acid

2-Hydroxybenzoic acid; $C_7H_6O_3$; relative molecular mass, 138

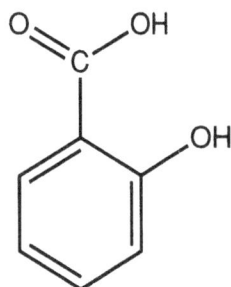

Salicylic acid is used topically to treat various dermatological disorders. It is the principal plasma metabolite of acetylsalicylic acid and can also arise from the metabolism of methyl salicylate and salicylamide. Salicylic acid is excreted in the urine, mostly as a conjugate with glycine (salicyluric acid).

The salicylic acid derivatives described below are commonly encountered drugs.

Acetylsalicylic acid

Aspirin; $C_9H_8O_4$; relative molecular mass, 180

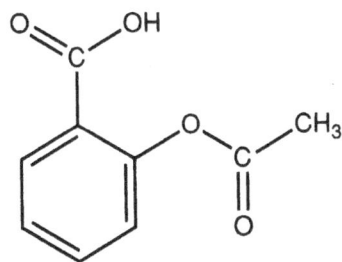

Acetylsalicylic acid is the most frequently used salicylic acid derivative. It is used as an analgesic and is also a metabolite of aloxiprin and benorilate. The estimated minimum lethal dose in an adult is 15 g.

Acetylsalicylic acid is rapidly metabolized by plasma esterases *in vivo* to salicylic acid, which is then excreted in the urine, mostly as a conjugate with glycine (salicyluric acid).

4-Aminosalicylic acid

p-Aminosalicylic acid; PAS; 4-amino-2-hydroxybenzoic acid; $C_7H_7NO_3$; relative molecular mass, 151

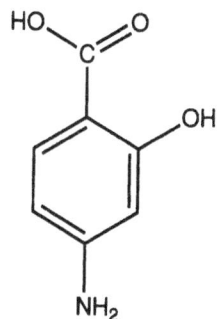

4-aminosalicylic acid is used in the treatment of tuberculosis.

Methyl salicylate

Methyl 2-hydroxybenzoate; salicylic acid methyl ester; $C_8H_8O_3$; relative molecular mass, 152

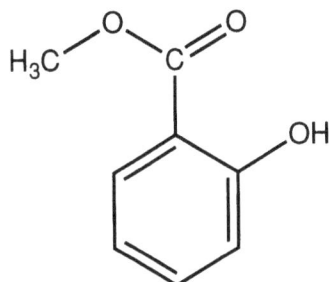

Methyl salicylate (oil of wintergreen) is a strong-smelling liquid at room temperature and is widely used in topical medicinal products. On ingestion it is more toxic than acetylsalicylic acid because it is more rapidly absorbed. Deaths have occurred in children after ingestion of as little as 4 ml; 30 ml is usually fatal in adults.

Methyl salicylate is partially metabolized to salicylic acid *in vivo*.

Salicylamide

2-Hydroxybenzamide; $C_7H_7NO_2$; relative molecular mass, 137

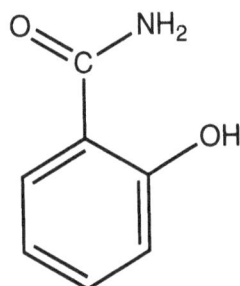

Salicylamide is used as an analgesic. On hydrolysis, it forms salicylic acid.

Salicylates give a distinctive purple colour with ferric ions and this reaction forms the basis of the test described. A simple dip-strip test for salicylates based on this reaction is available.

Acetylsalicylic acid and methyl salicylate do not themselves react with ferric ions, so that stomach contents and scene residues must be hydrolysed before analysis is performed. Salicylamide is only detectable after hydrolysis, even in urine samples.

Qualitative test

Applicable to urine, stomach contents and scene residues.

Reagent

Trinder's reagent. Mix 40 g of mercuric chloride dissolved in 850 ml of purified water with 120 ml of aqueous hydrochloric acid (1 mol/l) and 40 g of hydrated ferric nitrate, and dilute to 1 litre with purified water.

Method

Add 0.1 ml of Trinder's reagent to 2 ml of sample and mix for 5 seconds.

To test for acetylsalicylic acid or methyl salicylate in stomach contents or scene residues, and to test for salicylamide in urine, stomach contents or scene residues, first boil 1 ml of sample with 1 ml of aqueous hydrochloric acid (0.1 mol/l) for 10 minutes, cool, filter if necessary, and then neutralize with 1 ml of aqueous sodium hydroxide (0.1 mol/l).

Results

A strong violet colour indicates the presence of salicylates. Azide preservatives react strongly in this test, and weak false positives can be given by urine specimens containing high concentrations of ketones (ketone bodies).

This test is sensitive and will detect therapeutic dosage with salicylic acid, acetylsalicylic acid, 4-aminosalicylic acid, methyl salicylate and salicylamide.

Sensitivity

Salicylate, 10 mg/l.

Quantitative assay

Applicable to plasma or serum (1 ml).

Reagent

Trinder's reagent (see above).

Standards

Aqueous solutions containing salicylic acid at concentrations of 0, 200, 400 and 800 mg/l. Store at 4 °C when not in use.

Method

1. Add 5 ml of Trinder's reagent to 1 ml of sample or standard.
2. Vortex-mix for 30 seconds and centrifuge for 5 minutes.
3. Measure the absorbance of the supernatant at 540 nm against a plasma blank (see section 4.5.2).

Results

Calculate the plasma salicylate concentration from the graph obtained on analysis of the salicylate standards. Some salicylate metabolites interfere, but plasma concentrations of these compounds are usually low. Oxalates, for example, from fluoride/oxalate blood tubes, also interfere in this test.

Sensitivity

Salicylate, 50 mg/l.

Clinical interpretation

The topical use of salicylic acid and methyl salicylate and ingestion of salicylates may give rise to features of salicylism. Respiratory alkalosis followed by metabolic acidosis is characteristic, although in practice a mixed acid–base disturbance is usually seen. The results of blood gas analyses are an important guide to the severity of poisoning (see section

Fig. 13. Guide to the interpretation of plasma salicylate concentrations

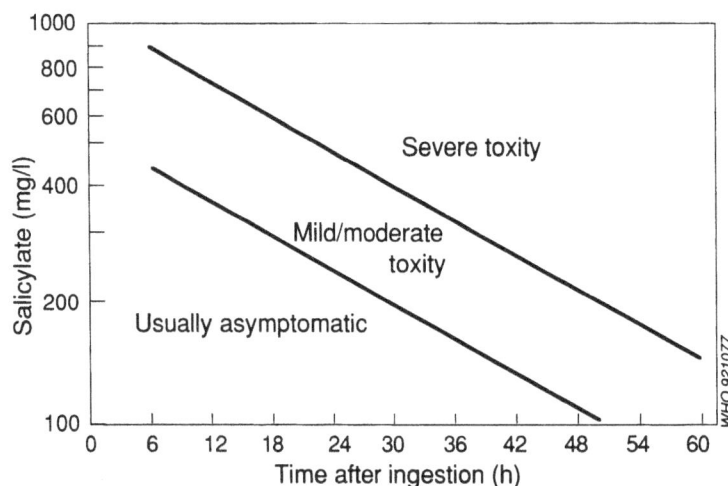

Results obtained within 6 hours of ingestion are unreliable and should be used with caution, since absorption may not be complete.

3.1.2). If acute poisoning is suspected, the plasma salicylate concentration should be measured using the method described above.

Active measures to correct acid–base status and urinary alkalinization to enhance elimination of the poison may be considered, depending on the patient's condition and the plasma salicylate concentration. Repeated oral activated charcoal may also be employed (see section 2.2.3).

Serial plasma salicylate and urine pH measurements are valuable in monitoring active treatment. A guide to the interpretation of plasma salicylate results is given in Fig. 13. Concentrations of up to 300 mg/l may be encountered during therapy in adults.

6.100 Strychnine

Strychnidin-10-one; $C_{21}H_{22}N_2O_2$; relative molecular mass, 334

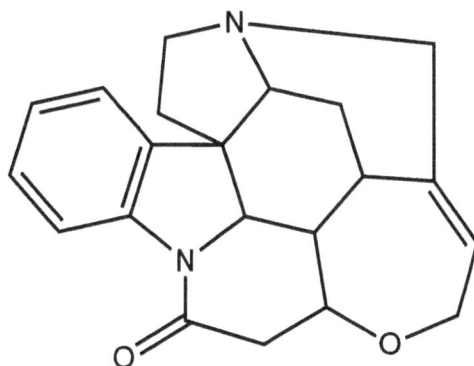

Strychnine and the related compound brucine (10,11-dimethoxystrychnine) are highly toxic alkaloids derived from the seeds of *Strychnos nux-vomica* and other *Strychnos* species. Strychnine has a bitter taste and is sometimes used in tonics for this reason. It is also used to exterminate rodents and other mammalian pests, and has been used to adulterate diamorphine (see section 6.73).

In addition to the simple tests given below, strychnine can be detected and differentiated from brucine by thin-layer chromatography of a basic or neutral extract of urine (see section 5.2.3).

Qualitative test
Applicable to stomach contents and scene residues.

Reagents

1. Concentrated ammonium hydroxide (relative density 0.88).
2. Ammonium vanadate (5 g/l) in concentrated sulfuric acid (relative density 1.83).

Method

1. Add 5 ml of sample to 1 ml of concentrated ammonium hydroxide and extract with 20 ml of chloroform for 10 minutes using a rotary mixer.
2. Centrifuge for 10 minutes, remove the upper, aqueous layer and transfer the solvent extract to a clean tube.
3. Evaporate the extract to dryness under a stream of compressed air or nitrogen and dissolve the residue in 100 μl of chloroform.
4. Transfer 50 μl of the reconstituted extract to a porcelain spotting tile and add 50 μl of ammonium vanadate solution.

Results

A violet colour which changes to red and then to yellow over 10 minutes suggests the presence of strychnine.

Sensitivity

Strychnine, 100 mg/l.

Confirmatory test

Applicable to stomach contents and scene residues.

Reagents

1. Granulated zinc.
2. Concentrated hydrochloric acid (relative density 1.18).
3. Aqueous sodium nitrite solution (100 g/l, freshly prepared).

Method

1. Add a granule of zinc to 1 ml of sample and 1 ml of concentrated hydrochloric acid and heat in a boiling water-bath for 10 minutes.
2. Cool, remove any remaining zinc and add 50 μl of sodium nitrite solution.

Results

Strychnine gives a pink colour.

Sensitivity

Strychnine, 10 mg/l.

Clinical interpretation

Ingestion of strychnine can cause convulsions and, notably, opisthotonos. Treatment is symptomatic and the patient may need intensive supportive care.

6.101 Sulfides

Sulfides such as sodium sulfide (Na$_2$S) and calcium sulfide (CaS) are used in depilatory agents, luminous paints, ore dressing and flotation, dye and plastics manufacture, photography, printing, veterinary medicine and a variety of other applications. Ingested elemental sulfur is metabolized to sulfide in the gastrointestinal tract; the ingestion of 10–20 g of sulfur may cause gastrointestinal symptoms. Hydrogen sulfide is often released when metallic sulfides are treated with water or acid, and their mammalian toxicity may be related to production of this compound.

Hydrogen sulfide (H$_2$S) is a colourless, extremely toxic gas which has, at low concentrations, an unpleasant odour of rotten eggs. At higher concentrations the olfactory response is lost and acute hydrogen sulfide poisoning is a leading cause of sudden death in the workplace. Hydrogen sulfide is released by decomposition of organic sulfur-containing materials and from sources of volcanic activity, and is used in the plastics, tanning, dye, rubber and petroleum industries, among others.

Hydrogen sulfide is rapidly metabolized *in vivo* by oxidation to sulfate and other pathways. Any analysis for sulfide in biological materials should be performed as quickly as possible, since the sulfide ion is unstable in such samples.

Qualitative test

Applicable to stomach contents and scene residues.

Reagents

1. Aqueous sulfuric acid (100 ml/l).
2. Lead acetate reagent. Mix 50 ml of lead acetate solution (100 g/l in boiled, purified water) and 5 ml of aqueous acetic acid (2 mol/l).

Method

1. Soak a strip of filter-paper in lead acetate reagent and allow to dry.
2. Add 3 ml of dilute sulfuric acid to 1 ml of sample, suspend the lead acetate-impregnated paper in the neck of the tube and place in a boiling water-bath **in a fume cupboard**.

Results

Sulfides give rise to hydrogen sulfide gas which blackens lead acetate paper.

Sensitivity

Sulfide, 50 mg/l.

There is no simple confirmatory test for sulfides; microdiffusion methods are unreliable.

Clinical interpretation

Exposure to hydrogen sulfide can give rise to headache, dizziness, drowsiness, nausea, sore throat, coma, convulsions, cardiac arrhythmias, respiratory depression and pulmonary oedema. Treatment may include the administration of 100% oxygen and nitrites.

6.102 Sulfites

Sulfites such as sodium sulfite (Na_2SO_3), sodium bisulfite ($NaHSO_3$), and sodium metabisulfite ($Na_2S_2O_3$) are used in the paper, water treatment, photographic and textile industries and as preservatives in beverages, foods and medications. Sulfur dioxide gas (SO_2) may be liberated on contact with acid. The estimated fatal dose of sodium sulfite in an adult is 10 g.

Quantitative assay

Applicable to urine.

Reagents

1. Magenta reagent. Add 0.02 g of basic magenta (fuchsine, CI 42510) to 100 ml of aqueous hydrochloric acid (1 mol/l) and store in the dark.
2. Formaldehyde solution. Dilute 1 ml of methanol-free aqueous form-aldehyde solution (340–380 g/kg) to 1 litre with purified water.

Standards

Anhydrous sodium sulfite (1.575 g) in 1 litre of purified water (to give a sulfite ion concentration of 1 g/l), diluted with purified water to give standards containing sulfite ion at concentrations of 0.5, 1.5, 3.0, 6.0 and 10.0 mg/l.

Method

1. Add 1 ml of magenta reagent and 3 ml of formaldehyde solution to 50 μl of sample.
2. Add 1 ml of magenta reagent and 3 ml of purified water to a second 50-μl portion of the sample.
3. Vortex-mix for 5 seconds and allow to stand for 5 minutes.
4. Measure the absorbance of the test solution from step 1 at 570 nm using the sample blank from step 2 as reference (see section 4.5.2).

Results

Construct a calibration graph following analysis of the standard sulfite solutions and calculate the sulfite concentration in the sample.

Sensitivity

Sulfite, 0.5 mg/l.

Clinical interpretation

Acute sulfite poisoning can cause generalized flush, faintness, syncope, wheezing, shortness of breath, cyanosis and cold skin. Urticaria and angioedema may be seen within minutes of exposure, and may be followed by acute bronchospasm and respiratory arrest in certain people. Treatment is symptomatic and supportive. The normal urinary concentration of sulfite ion is less than 6 mg/l.

6.103 Tetrachloroethylene

Perchlorethylene; tetrachloroethene; $CCl_2{:}CCl_2$; relative molecular mass, 166

Tetrachloroethylene is used as an anthelminthic and as a solvent in dry-cleaning and vapour degreasing. Acute poisoning with this compound is normally from massive accidental exposure or deliberate inhalation (solvent abuse). Only about 0.5% of an absorbed dose of tetrachloroethylene is metabolized to trichloroacetic acid, but this can be detected in urine using the Fujiwara test.

Qualitative test

Applicable to urine. Fujiwara test — see carbon tetrachloride monograph (section 6.23).

Results

An intense red/purple colour in the upper, pyridine layer indicates the presence of trichloro compounds. The blank analysis excludes contamination with chloroform from the laboratory atmosphere.

This test will detect ingestion or exposure to low doses of compounds that are extensively metabolized to trichloroacetic acid, such as chloral hydrate, dichloralphenazone and trichloroethylene, 12–24 hours later. With tetrachloroethylene, the test is correspondingly less sensitive, since such a small proportion of a dose is metabolized.

Sensitivity

Trichloroacetate, 1 mg/l.

Clinical interpretation

Signs of poisoning with tetrachloroethylene include ataxia, nausea, vomiting, coma, respiratory depression and cardiac arrhythmias.

Hepatorenal damage is very uncommon. Treatment is symptomatic and supportive.

6.104 Thallium

Thallium (Tl) salts are employed in the manufacture of semiconductors, pigments and lenses, and are used as rodenticides in many countries. The lethal dose of thallium in an adult is 0.2–1 g.

The test given below can be used to give an approximate measure of urinary thallium concentration if poisoning with this element is suspected.

Quantitative assay
Applicable to urine.

Reagents

1. Cyanide reagent. Dissolve 1.6 g of sodium hydroxide, 1.2 g of potassium sodium tartrate and 1.36 g of potassium cyanide in 10 ml of water. **Take care when using concentrated cyanide solutions.**
2. Dithizone solution (250 mg/l) in chloroform (freshly prepared).

Standards

Blank urine to which has been added a solution of thallium acetate in purified water (1.0-g/l) to give thallium ion concentrations of 0.1, 1.0, 5.0 and 10.0 mg/l.

Method

1. Add 1 ml of cyanide reagent to 5 ml of sample or standard in a 10-ml glass-stoppered test-tube and vortex-mix for 10 sec onds.
2. Add 2 ml of dithizone solution, vortex-mix for 1 minute, and centrifuge for 5 minutes.
3. Discard the upper, aqueous layer and filter the chloroform extract through phase-separating filter-paper into a clean tube.
4. Measure the absorbance of the extract at 480 nm against a blank urine extract (see section 4.5.2).

Results

A pink/red colour in the lower chloroform layer indicates the presence of thallium at concentrations of 1 mg/l or more. Construct a calibration graph of absorbance against thallium concentration in the standards and measure the thallium concentration in the sample. A number of metal ions may interfere in this assay. Atomic absorption spectrophotometry is needed in order to measure thallium definitively.

Sensitivity
Thallium, 0.1 mg/l.

Clinical interpretation

Acute poisoning with thallium salts may lead to gastrointestinal stasis, while intermediate and late effects may include disturbances of the peripheral and central nervous systems, the cardiorespiratory system, eyes and skin. Scalp and facial hair loss is a typical sign of thallium poisoning. Patients with urinary thallium concentrations exceeding 0.5 mg/l should be treated with potassium ferrohexacyanoferrate (Prussian blue; see Table 6) until urinary thallium excretion is below 0.5 mg/day.

6.105 Theophylline

1,3-Dimethylxanthine; $C_7H_8N_4O_2$; relative molecular mass, 180

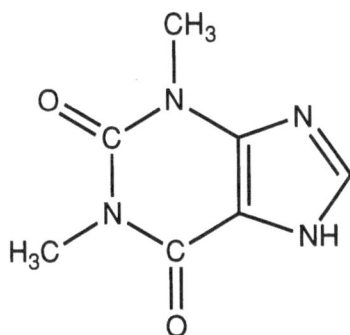

Theophylline is a bronchodilator widely used in the treatment of asthma, often as a mixture with ethylenediamine (aminophylline). Theophylline is metabolized to 3-methylxanthine, 1,3-dimethyluric acid, and 1-methuric acid; caffeine is a metabolite in neonates.

There is no simple test for theophylline applicable to biological fluids. Ethylenediamine gives a green colour in the *o*-cresol/ammonia urine test used to detect paracetamol, but in this case only indicates prior ingestion of aminophylline (see section 6.83).

Quantitative assay

Applicable to plasma or serum.

Reagents

1. Tris buffer (0.2 mol/l, pH 7.0). Mix 200 ml of aqueous hydrochloric acid (1 mol/l) and 214 ml of aqueous tris(hydroxymethyl)amino-methane free base (121 g/l).
2. Sodium carbonate buffer (0.1 mol/l, pH 9.0). Mix 10 ml of aqueous sodium carbonate (10.6 g/l) and 890 ml of aqueous sodium bicarbonate solution (8.4 g/l).

Standards

Solutions containing theophylline concentrations of 5, 10, 20 and 50 mg/l in blank plasma.

Method

1. Add 0.5 ml of tris buffer to 2.0 ml of sample or standard, and add 10 ml of chloroform.
2. Vortex-mix for 2 minutes, and centrifuge for 5 minutes.
3. Remove the upper, aqueous layer and filter 8 ml of the chloroform extract through phase-separating filter-paper into a clean tube.
4. Add 2.5 ml of sodium carbonate buffer to the chloroform extract, vortex-mix for 2 minutes and centrifuge for 5 minutes.
5. Transfer 2.0 ml of the aqueous extract (upper layer) to a quartz spectrophotometer cell and measure the absorbance at 280 nm against a plasma blank (see section 4.5.2).

Results

Construct a calibration graph following analysis of the standard theophylline solutions and calculate the theophylline concentration in the sample. Specimens containing a theophylline concentration of more than 50 mg/l should be diluted with blank plasma and re-analysed.

Use of the pH 9.0 extraction and measurement at 280 nm minimizes interference from barbiturates, but caffeine, theophylline metabolites and some other drugs may interfere in this assay.

Sensitivity

Theophylline, 5 mg/l.

Clinical interpretation

Acute overdosage with theophylline and other xanthines may cause palpitations, hypotension, diuresis, central nervous system stimulation, nausea, vomiting, marked hypokalaemia, metabolic acidosis and convulsions. Treatment is normally symptomatic and supportive, with particular emphasis on correcting the hypokalaemia. Repeat-dose oral activated charcoal can be used to enhance theophylline clearance (see section 2.2.3).

Plasma theophylline concentrations attained during therapy are normally less than 20 mg/l. Toxic effects are more frequent at concentrations above 30 mg/l, while plasma concentrations of 50 mg/l or more may be encountered in fatal cases.

6.106 Thiocyanates

Potassium thiocyanate (KSCN) and sodium thiocyanate (NaSCN) were previously used in the treatment of hypertension, but nowadays these compounds are used principally as synthetic intermediates, and in the printing, dye and photographic industries. Thiocyanate is a metabolite of cyanide and thiocyanate toxicity is most commonly encountered as a result of chronic sodium nitroprusside administration. Thiocyanate is also found in the blood of cigarette smokers from metabolism of cyanide. Thiocyanate is excreted in urine; the plasma half-life is about 3 days if renal function is normal.

Qualitative test
Applicable to urine, stomach contents and scene residues.

Reagent
Aqueous ferric chloride solution (50 g/l).

Method
Add 0.1 ml of ferric chloride solution to 0.1 ml of sample and mix.

Results
A deep red colour indicates the presence of thiocyanate.

Sensitivity
Thiocyanate, 50 mg/l.

Quantitative assay
Applicable to plasma or serum.

Reagents
1. Aqueous trichloroacetic acid solution (50 g/l).
2. Ferric nitrate reagent. Dissolve 80 g of ferric nitrate nona-hydrate in 250 ml of aqueous nitric acid (2 mol/l), dilute to 500 ml with purified water and filter.

Standards

Prepare aqueous solutions containing thiocyanate ion concentrations of 5, 10, 20, 50 and 100 mg/l by dilution from an aqueous solution of potassium thiocyanate (1.67 g/l, equivalent to a thiocyanate ion concentration of 1.00 g/l).

Method

1. Add 4.5 ml of trichloroacetic acid solution to 0.5 ml of sample or standard, vortex-mix for 30 seconds and centrifuge for 5 minutes.
2. In a darkened room, add 2 ml of the supernatant to 4 ml of ferric nitrate reagent, vortex-mix for 5 seconds, and measure the absorbance at 460 nm against a reagent blank (see section 4.5.2).

Results

Construct a calibration graph following analysis of the standard thiocyanate solutions and calculate the thiocyanate concentration in the sample.

Sensitivity

Thiocyanate, 2 mg/l.

Clinical interpretation

Acute ingestion of thiocyanate salts may cause disorientation, weakness, hypotension, confusion, psychotic behaviour, muscular spasm and convulsions. Treatment is normally symptomatic and supportive.

In nonsmokers, plasma thiocyanate concentrations range from 0.1 to 0.4 mg/l, while in heavy smokers concentrations typically range from 5 to 20 mg/l. Plasma thiocyanate concentrations can reach 100 mg/l during sodium nitroprusside therapy, but toxicity often occurs at concentrations above 120 mg/l. Plasma concentrations of the order of 200 mg/l have been reported in fatalities.

6.107 Tin

Metallic tin (Sn) and its inorganic salts are used in metallurgy and in tanning, polishing and metal coating ("tin" cans). Organotin compounds, usually ethyl, butyl or phenyl derivatives, such as tributyl tin, are used as pesticides, in antifouling paints on ships, and as stabilizers in plastics. Inorganic tin compounds are poorly absorbed after ingestion, but organotin derivatives are well absorbed from the gastrointestinal tract and can cause serious systemic toxicity.

There are no simple qualitative tests for either inorganic tin or organotin compounds suitable for use in the diagnosis of acute poisoning.

Clinical interpretation

Ingestion of high doses of inorganic tin compounds may cause nausea, vomiting and diarrhoea. Acute exposure to organotin derivatives may cause headache, vomiting, abdominal pain, tinnitus, deafness, loss of memory, disorientation, coma and respiratory depression. Treatment is symptomatic and supportive.

6.108 Tolbutamide

1-Butyl-3-*p*-tolylsulfonylurea; $C_{12}H_{18}N_2O_3S$; relative molecular mass, 270

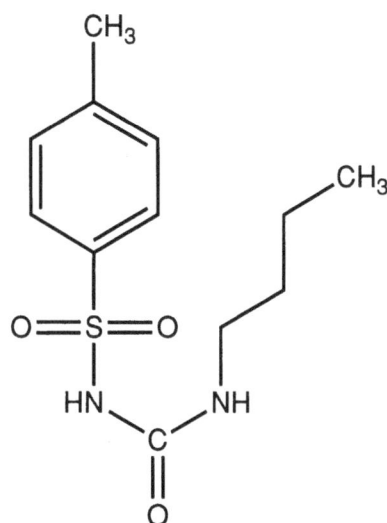

Tolbutamide is a hypoglycaemic agent widely used to treat diabetes. About 85% of an oral dose is excreted in urine as the 4-carboxy and 4-hydroxymethyl metabolites; only about 5% is excreted unchanged. The normal dose of this drug is up to 3 g/day; a fatality has followed the ingestion of 50 g of tolbutamide.

There is no simple qualitative test for tolbutamide in biological specimens. However, the colorimetric procedure given below can be used to assess the severity of poisoning if overdosage is suspected. This method can also be used to measure other sulfonylurea hypoglycaemic agents, such as chlorpropamide and acetohexamide, in plasma using the appropriate standards.

Quantitative assay

Applicable to plasma or serum.

Reagents

1. Aqueous hydrochloric acid (0.02 mol/l).
2. Fluorodinitrobenzene reagent. 1-Fluoro-2,4-dinitrobenzene (1 g/l) in *iso*-amyl acetate, freshly prepared.

Standards

Solutions containing tolbutamide concentrations of 20, 50, 100 and 200 mg/l in blank plasma.

Method

1. Add 2.5 ml of dilute hydrochloric acid to 0.5 ml of sample or standard and add 10 ml of *iso*-amyl acetate.
2. Vortex-mix for 2 minutes and centrifuge for 5 minutes.
3. Transfer 6 ml of the upper, organic layer to a clean tube, add 1 ml of fluorodinitrobenzene reagent and vortex-mix for 30 seconds.
4. Place a loosely fitting glass cap on the top of the tube and heat on a boiling water-bath for 10 minutes.
5. Cool, allow to stand at room temperature for 30 minutes, and measure the absorbance at 346 nm against a plasma blank (see section 4.5.2).

Results

Construct a calibration graph following analysis of the standard tolbutamide solutions and calculate the tolbutamide concentration in the sample. Samples containing tolbutamide at concentrations above 200 mg/l should be diluted with blank plasma and re-analysed.

The chromogenic reagent used in this test reacts with most primary and secondary amines and some other functional groups. The results must therefore be interpreted with caution if other drugs may be present.

Sensitivity

Tolbutamide, 10 mg/l.

Clinical interpretation

Overdosage with sulfonylurea hypoglycaemics such as tolbutamide may cause nausea, vomiting, abdominal pain, hypotension, drowsiness, prolonged hypoglycaemia, hyperkalaemia, metabolic acidosis, coma, convulsions, pulmonary oedema and circulatory failure. Treatment includes correction of hypoglycaemia by giving glucose.

Plasma tolbutamide concentrations attained during therapy are normally 40–100 mg/l and toxicity may be expected at plasma concentrations above 200 mg/l. Measurement of blood glucose is important in establishing the diagnosis of poisoning with tolbutamide and other hypoglycaemic drugs and in monitoring treatment (see section 3.1.1).

6.109 Toluene

Methylbenzene; $C_6H_5.CH_3$; relative molecular mass, 92

Toluene is used as a solvent in adhesives, paints and paint-strippers (which often also contain dichloromethane or methanol) and is widely used in industry. Acute toluene poisoning is normally from massive accidental exposure or deliberate inhalation (glue sniffing, solvent abuse). Some 80% of a dose of toluene is metabolized to benzoic acid, which is conjugated with glycine to give hippuric acid. Measurement of urinary hippurate excretion can be used as an index of chronic toluene exposure, but sodium benzoate or benzoic acid used as food preservatives are also metabolized to hippurate and results should therefore be interpreted with caution.

Quantitative assay
Applicable to urine.

Reagents
1. Aqueous hydrochloric acid (0.05 mol/l).
2. Dimethylaminobenzaldehyde reagent. *p*-Dimethylaminobenzaldehyde (40 g/l) in acetic anhydride containing a few crystals (about 0.5 g) of anhydrous sodium acetate.
3. Sodium chloride (solid).
4. Precipitated silica.

Standards
Blank urine, plus urine to which hippuric acid has been added to give concentrations of 0.2, 0.5, 1.0 and 2.0 g/l. All samples must be prepared from one urine specimen. These solutions are stable for 1 month if stored at 4 °C in the dark.

Method
1. Adjust the pH of 1.0 ml of sample or standard to 2 with dilute hydrochloric acid, and add sodium chloride until the solution is saturated.

2. Add 2 ml of diethyl ether : methanol (9:1), vortex-mix for 1 minute and centrifuge for 5 minutes.
3. Aspirate the upper, ether layer into a clean tube and re-extract the aqueous phase with a further 2 ml of diethyl ether : methanol (9:1).
4. Combine the ethereal extracts and add 1 ml to about 0.5 g of precipitated silica in a clean tube.
5. Remove the solvent under a stream of compressed air or nitrogen, add 3 ml of dimethylaminobenzaldehyde reagent, and heat on a heating block at 135 °C for 5 minutes.
6. Cool, add 4 ml of methanol, vortex-mix for 1 minute and centrifuge for 5 minutes.
7. Aspirate the methanolic extract into a clean tube and re-extract the silica with a further 4 ml of methanol.
8. Combine the methanolic extracts and measure the absorbance at 460 nm against the blank urine extract (see section 4.5.2).

Results

Prepare a calibration graph following analysis of the standard hippuric acid solutions and calculate the hippuric acid concentration in the sample. It is important to use a portion of the same urine used to prepare the standards as the blank, since hippurate excretion varies with dietary benzoate intake, as indicated above.

Sensitivity

Hippurate, 0.1 g/l.

Clinical interpretation

Features of acute toluene poisoning include ataxia, nausea, vomiting, respiratory depression, coma and cardiac arrhythmia. Hepatorenal damage is uncommon. Treatment is symptomatic and supportive.

Urinary hippuric acid concentrations are normally 0.1–0.2 g/l; concentrations greater than 1 g/l indicate prior exposure to toluene if other possible sources of benzoate can be excluded. In acute poisoning with toluene, death may supervene before hippurate excretion is raised.

6.110 1,1,1-Trichloroethane

Methylchloroform; $CCl_3.CH_3$; relative molecular mass, 133

1,1,1-Trichloroethane is widely used as a solvent for dry-cleaning and vapour degreasing, and in typewriter correction fluids. Acute poisoning with 1,1,1-trichloroethane is normally from massive accidental exposure or deliberate inhalation (solvent abuse). Some 2% of an absorbed dose of

1,1,1-trichloroethane is metabolized to 2,2,2-trichloroethanol and then to trichloroacetic acid. This can be detected in urine using the Fujiwara test.

Qualitative test

Applicable to urine. Fujiwara test — see carbon tetrachloride monograph (section 6.23).

Results

An intense red/purple colour in the upper, pyridine layer indicates the presence of trichloro compounds. The blank analysis excludes contamination with chloroform from the laboratory atmosphere.

This test is sensitive and will detect ingestion or exposure to low doses of compounds that are extensively metabolized to trichloroacetic acid, such as chloral hydrate, dichloralphenazone and trichloroethylene, 12–24 hours later. However, with 1,1,1-trichloroethane the test is correspondingly less sensitive, since such a small proportion of a dose is metabolized.

Sensitivity

Trichloroacetate, 1 mg/l.

Clinical interpretation

Signs of poisoning with 1,1,1-trichloroethane include ataxia, nausea, vomiting, coma, respiratory depression and cardiac arrhythmias. Hepatorenal damage is uncommon. Treatment is symptomatic and supportive.

6.111 Trichloroethylene

Trichloroethene; CHCl:CCl$_2$; relative molecular mass, 131

Trichloroethylene is a well known solvent and has also been used as a general anaesthetic. Acute poisoning with trichloroethylene is normally from massive accidental exposure or deliberate inhalation (solvent abuse). As with some hypnotic drugs, including chloral hydrate and dichloralphenazone, trichloroethylene is extensively metabolized (about 80% of an absorbed dose) to trichloroacetic acid. This can be detected in urine using the Fujiwara test.

Qualitative test

Applicable to urine. Fujiwara test — see carbon tetrachloride monograph (section 6.23).

Results

An intense red/purple colour in the upper, pyridine layer indicates the presence of trichloro compounds. The blank analysis excludes contamination with chloroform from the laboratory atmosphere.

This test is very sensitive and will detect exposure to trichloroethylene 12–24 hours later. However, other compounds also give rise to trichloroacetic acid *in vivo*, including the chlorinated solvents 1,1,1-trichloroethane and tetrachloroethylene, and caution must be exercised in reporting results.

Sensitivity

Trichloroacetate, 1 mg/l.

Clinical interpretation

Clinical features of acute poisoning with trichloroethylene include ataxia, nausea, vomiting, coma, respiratory depression and cardiac arrhythmias. Hepatorenal damage may also occur. Treatment is symptomatic and supportive.

6.112 Verapamil

5-(*N*-(3,4-Dimethoxyphenethyl)-*N*-methylamino)-2-(3,4-dimethoxyphenyl)-2-isopropylvaleronitrile; $C_{27}H_{38}N_2O_4$; relative molecular mass, 455

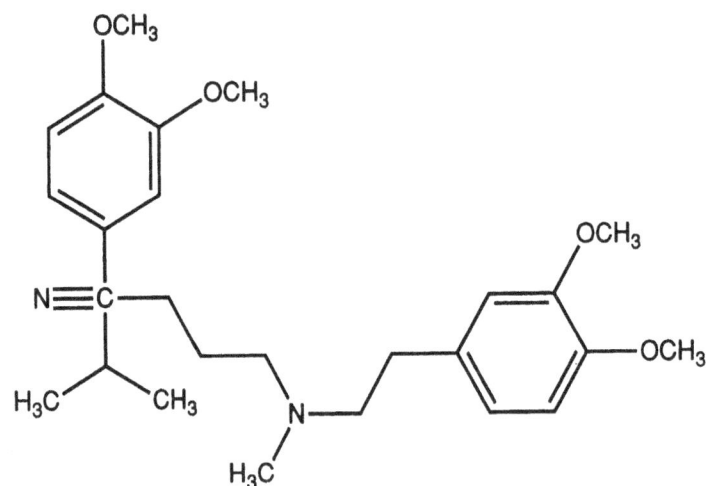

Verapamil is used to treat hypertension. Metabolic pathways include *N*-dealkylation (*N*-demethylation gives norverapamil which is pharmacologically active) with *O*-demethylation and conjugation of the resulting compounds. About 70% of a dose is excreted in urine, 10% as norverapamil, and less than 5% as the parent compound.

There is no simple qualitative test for verapamil, but this compound and its metabolites can be detected and identified by thin-layer chromatography of a basic solvent extract of urine (see section 5.2.3).

Clinical interpretation

Acute ingestion of verapamil may cause bradycardia, hypotension, cardiac arrhythmia, metabolic acidosis, hyperglycaemia, coma and gastrointestinal haemorrhage. Treatment is supportive, and may include the administration of calcium salts and inotropic agents in severe cases.

6.113 Zinc

Zinc (Zn) is used in some alloys (brass), in metal plating (galvanizing) and in many other applications. Finely divided zinc chloride ($ZnCl_2$) is produced by chemical smoke generators and this compound is also used in soldering flux, dry battery cells and dental cement. Zinc oxide (ZnO) is used in making pharmaceuticals (zinc oxide plaster), rubber and white pigments. The acute oral toxicity of compounds like zinc chloride is limited since they are powerful emetics. Fatalities have been reported after the intravenous administration of 7.4 g of zinc and the inhalation of zinc chloride fumes.

There is no simple qualitative or quantitative test for zinc in biological specimens.

Clinical interpretation

Acute poisoning with zinc compounds may cause fever, nausea, vomiting, diarrhoea, lethargy, muscle aches, weakness, cyanosis, pulmonary oedema, acute pancreatitis and acute renal failure. Treatment is symptomatic and supportive.

Bibliography

Section 1. General considerations

Baselt RC, Cravey RH. *Disposition of toxic drugs and chemicals in man*, 3rd ed. Chicago, Year Book Medical, 1990.

Basic tests for pharmaceutical dosage forms. Geneva, World Health Organization, 1991.

Basic tests for pharmaceutical substances. Geneva, World Health Organization, 1986.

Duffus JH. Glossary for chemists of terms used in toxicology. *Pure and applied chemistry*, 1993, **65** : 2003–2122.

International Union of Pure and Applied Chemistry/International Programme on Chemical Safety. *Chemical safety matters.* Cambridge, Cambridge University Press, 1992.

Moffat AC, ed. *Clarke's isolation and identification of drugs*, 2nd ed. London, Pharmaceutical Press, 1986.

Section 2. Clinical aspects of analytical toxicology

Dreisbach RH, Robertson WO. *Handbook of poisoning: prevention, diagnosis and treatment*, 12th ed. Norwalk, CT, Appleton Lange, 1987.

Ellenhorn MJ, Barceloux DG. *Medical toxicology: diagnosis and treatment of human poisoning.* Amsterdam, Elsevier, 1988.

Goldfrank LR et al., ed. *Goldfrank's toxicologic emergencies*, 4th ed. Norwalk, CT, Appleton Lange, 1990.

Haddad LM, Winchester JF, ed. *Clinical management of poisoning and drug overdose*, 2nd ed. Philadelphia, Saunders, 1990.

Meredith TJ et al., ed. *Naloxone, flumazenil and dantrolene as antidotes.* Cambridge, Cambridge University Press, 1993 (IPCS/CEC Evaluation of Antidotes Series, Vol. 1).

Meredith TJ et al., ed. *Antidotes for poisoning by cyanide.* Cambridge, Cambridge University Press, 1993 (IPCS/CEC Evaluation of Antidotes Series, Vol. 2).

Meredith TJ et al., ed. *Antidotes for poisoning by paracetamol.* Cambridge, Cambridge University Press, 1994 (IPCS/CEC Evaluation of Antidotes Series, Vol. 3).

Proudfoot AT. *Acute poisoning diagnosis and management,* 2nd ed. Oxford, Butterworth Heinemann, 1993.

Section 3. General laboratory findings in clinical toxicology

Walmsley RN, White GH. *A guide to diagnostic clinical chemistry.* London, Blackwell, 1983.

Whitehead TP et al. *Clinical chemistry and haematology: adult reference values.* London, BUPA, 1994.

Section 4. Practical aspects of analytical toxicology

Anderson R. *Sample pretreatment and separation.* Chichester, Wiley, 1987 (Analytical chemistry by open learning (ACOL) series).

Denney RC, Sinclair R. *Visible and ultraviolet spectroscopy.* Chichester, Wiley, 1987 (Analytical chemistry by open learning (ACOL) series).

Feldstein L, Klendhoj NC. The determination of volatile substances by micro-diffusion analysis. *Journal of forensic sciences,* 1957, **2**:39–58.

Hamilton RJ, Hamilton S. *Thin layer chromatography.* Chichester, Wiley, 1987 (Analytical chemistry by open learning (ACOL) series).

Hawcroft D, Hector T. *Clinical specimens.* Chichester, Wiley, 1987 (Analytical chemistry by open learning (ACOL) series).

Sewell P, Clarke B. *Chromatographic separations.* Chichester, Wiley, 1987 (Analytical chemistry by open learning (ACOL) series).

Woodget BW, Cooper D. *Samples and standards.* Chichester, Wiley, 1987 (Analytical chemistry by open learning (ACOL) series).

Section 5. Qualitative tests for poisons

DFG-TIAFT. *Thin layer chromatographic R_f values of toxicologically relevant substances on standardised systems,* 2nd ed. Weinheim, VCH, 1992.

Stead AH et al. Standardised thin-layer chromatographic systems for the identification of drugs and poisons. *Analyst (London),* 1982, **107**:1106–1168.

Section 6. Monographs — analytical and toxicological data

Budavari S, ed. *The Merck index*, 11th ed. Rahway, NJ, Merck, 1989.

Fiegel F, Anger V. *Spot tests in organic analysis*, 7th ed. Amsterdam, Elsevier, 1966.

Fiegel F, Anger V. *Spot tests in inorganic analysis*, 6th ed. Amsterdam, Elsevier, 1972.

Friberg GF et al. ed. *Handbook on the toxicology of metals*, 2nd ed. Vol. I and II. Amsterdam, Elsevier, 1986.

Hayes WJ, Laws ER, ed. *Handbook of pesticide toxicology*, Vols 1–3. San Diego, Academic Press, 1991.

Lenga RE. *The Sigma Aldrich library of chemical safety data*, 2nd ed. Vols 1 and 2. Milwaukee, Sigma Aldrich, 1988.

Reynolds JEF, ed. *Martindale. The extra pharmacopoeia*, 30th ed. London, Pharmaceutical Press, 1993.

Richardson ML, Gangolis S, ed. *The dictionary of substances and their effects.* Cambridge, Royal Society of Chemistry, 1992.

Schutz H. *Benzodiazepines: a handbook.* Berlin, Springer Verlag, 1982.

Schutz H. *Dünnschicht-chromatographische Suchanalyse für 1,4-Benzodiazepine in Harn, Blut und Mageninhalt.* [*Thin-layer chromatographic screening analysis for 1,4-benzodiazepines in urine, blood and stomach contents.*] Weinheim, VCH, 1986.

The agrochemicals handbook, 3rd ed. Cambridge, Royal Society of Chemistry, 1991.

Weast RC, ed. *Handbook of chemistry and physics*, 70th ed. Boca Raton, CRC Press, 1989.

Worthing CR, ed. *The pesticide manual*, 9th ed. Thornton Heath, British Crop Protection Council, 1991.

Glossary

This glossary is included to aid communication between the toxicologist and the clinician. The definitions given refer to the use of terms in this book, and are not necessarily valid in other contexts.

Abortifacient   A means of causing abortion.

Abuse   Excessive or improper use of drugs or other substances.

Abuse, volatile substance   The intentional inhalation of volatile substances, such as organic solvents or aerosol propellants, with the aim of achieving intoxication.

Acetylcholine   The main neurotransmitter of the vertebrate and invertebrate peripheral nervous systems (*see also*: Anticholinergic, Cholinergic).

Acetylcholinesterase   Acetylcholine acetylhydrolase, EC 3.1.1.7. Enzyme that hydrolyses the neurotransmitter acetylcholine within the central nervous system (*see also*: Cholinesterase).

Acidosis   Pathological condition resulting from accumulation of acid in, or loss of base from, the blood or body tissues.

Acidosis, lactic   Metabolic acidosis due to the production of excessive amounts of lactic acid.

Acidosis, metabolic   Acidosis of metabolic origin.

Acidosis, respiratory   Acidosis of respiratory origin.

Acne   Inflammation in or around the sebaceous glands, generally of the face, chest and back.

Acute   Sudden or short-term (cf. Chronic).

Acute-on-chronic   Describes a sudden episode of increased severity against a background of prolonged disease or exposure.

β-Adrenoceptor blocking agent   See β-Blocker.

Agonist   Drug that has affinity for, and stimulates physiological activity at, cell receptors (cf. Antagonist).

β-Agonist   Agent exerting an agonist effect at a *β*-adrenoceptor.

Agranulocytosis   A blood disorder in which there is an absence of granulocytes.

Akathisia   An inability to sit still.

Albuminuria   The presence of albumin in the urine.

Alkaline diuresis   Technique for rendering the urine alkaline, for example, by intravenous administration of sodium bicarbonate, to enhance excretion of certain acidic poisons such as salicylate.

Alkalinization   To add alkali or to make alkaline.

Alkaloid   A nitrogenous organic compound of plant origin.

Alkalosis   Pathological condition resulting from accumulation of base in, or loss of acid from, the blood or body tissues.

Anaemia   Deficiency of erythrocytes or of haemoglobin in the blood.

Anaesthetic   A substance producing either local or general loss of sensation.

Analgesic   A substance that relieves pain, without producing anaesthesia or loss of consciousness.

Anaphylaxis   Reaction to foreign material as a result of increased susceptibility following previous exposure.

Angioedema   Marked swelling of body tissues.

Anion gap   In blood plasma, the difference between the concentration of sodium and the sum of the concentrations of chloride and bicarbonate.

Anorexia   Lack or loss of appetite for food (cf. Bulimia).

Anoxia   Absence or lack of oxygen.

Antagonist   An agent that reverses or reduces the pharmacological action of a second agent.

Anthelminthic   An agent that kills intestinal worms.

Antiarrhythmic   An agent used to treat a cardiac arrhythmia.

Antibiotic   An agent produced or derived from a microorganism used to control or kill other microorganisms.

Antibody   A protein produced in the body in response to exposure to an antigen; it recognizes and specifically binds the antigen.

Anticholinergic   An antagonist to the neurotransmitter acetylcholine.

Anticoagulant   A drug that prevents clotting of blood.

Anticonvulsant   A drug used to control epilepsy.

Antidepressant   A drug used to treat depression.

Antidiabetic   A drug used to treat diabetes mellitus.

Antidote   An agent that neutralizes or opposes the action of a poison on an organism.

Antigen   Any substance that stimulates the body to produce an antibody.

Antihistamine   An antagonist to histamine.

Anti-inflammatory   Reducing or preventing inflammation.

Anti-knock agent   A substance, such as tetra-ethyl lead, used to prevent pre-ignition (knock) in internal combustion engines.

Antipsychotic   A drug used to treat psychosis.

Antipyretic   A drug that relieves or reduces fever.

Antiseptic   An agent used to control or kill microorganisms.

Anuria   Complete absence of urine production (cf. Oliguria, Polyuria).

Apathy   Indifference.

Apnoea   Cessation of breathing.

Areflexia   Generalized absence of reflexes.

Arrhythmia   Any variation from the normal rhythm of the heartbeat.

Aspiration   (i) The act of withdrawing a fluid by suction. (ii) The breathing in of a foreign body, e.g. vomit.

Asthma   Chronic respiratory disease characterized by wheezing and difficulty in breathing out.

Ataxia   Failure of muscular coordination.

Bilirubin   A pigment, derived from the breakdown of haemoglobin, that occurs in soluble form in blood and in bile.

239

Biological specimens   Samples of tissues (including blood, hair), secretions (breast milk, saliva, sweat), excretion products (bile, urine) and other material such as stomach contents or vomit derived from a patient.

Blank   Used in analytical chemistry to denote a specimen not containing the analyte of interest and from which a background reading can be obtained.

β-Blocker   Agent inhibiting the action of endogenous neurotransmitters (epinephrine, norepinephrine) at *β*-adrenoceptors.

Bradyarrhythmia   Arrhythmia associated with an excessively slow heartbeat (cf. Tachyarrhythmia).

Bradycardia   Excessively slow heartbeat (cf. Tachycardia).

Bronchoconstriction   Narrowing of the bronchial tubes.

Bronchodilation   Expansion of the bronchial tubes.

Bronchorrhoea   Abnormally copious mucous discharge from the walls of the bronchial tubes.

Bronchospasm   Intermittent, violent contraction of the walls of the bronchial tubes.

Bulimia   Morbid hunger (cf. Anorexia).

Butyrophenones   A group of antipsychotic drugs.

Carboxyhaemoglobin   Product formed when carbon monoxide binds to haemoglobin.

Cardiogenic   Produced in, or originating from, the heart.

Cardiotoxic   Having a harmful effect on the action of the heart.

Catheterization   Introduction of a tube for adding or removing fluids to or from the body.

Caustic   Having a corrosive action on skin and flesh.

Cerebellar   Relating to the hind part of the brain concerned with voluntary movement and balance.

Cerebral   Relating to the brain.

Chelate   Compound in which a central metallic ion is attached to an organic molecule (chelating agent) at two or more positions (*see also*: Sequestrant).

Chelating agent   A compound capable of forming a chelate with a metal ion.

Chelation therapy Treatment with a chelating agent to enhance the elimination or reduce the toxicity of a poison.

Cholinergic Stimulated, activated or transmitted by acetylcholine.

Cholinesterase Enzyme (E.C. 3.1.1.8) that catalyses the breakdown of a choline ester to choline (*see also*: Acetylcholinesterase).

Chorea Irregular, involuntary movements of the limbs or face.

Chronic Long-term (cf. Acute).

Cirrhosis Wasting disease of the liver accompanied by abnormal growth of connective tissue (scar tissue).

Coagulopathy Disorder of blood clotting.

Colic Severe, intermittent pain associated with the abdomen.

Conjugate Metabolite formed by covalent bonding with, for example, glucuronic acid, sulfate, acetate, or glycine.

Conjunctiva The outer surface of the eyeball and the inner surface of the eyelid.

Conjunctivitis Inflammation of the conjunctiva.

Contaminant An impurity.

Corrosive Able to eat away or dissolve by chemical action.

Cosmetic Concerned with improving appearance or hygiene.

Cross-contamination Accidental introduction of an impurity.

Crystalluria Presence of crystals in the urine.

Cutaneous Associated with the skin.

Cyanosis Blue appearance, especially of the skin and mucous membranes, due to deficient oxygenation.

Deamination Removal of an amine from a molecule.

Delirium State characterized by hallucinations, disorientation, and restlessness.

Delirium tremens Clinical features associated with alcohol withdrawal (*see also*: Withdrawal, drug).

Denature (i) To alter the physical nature of a substance or mixture. (ii) To render unfit for human consumption.

Depigmentation   Loss of natural coloration.

Depilatory agent   A substance applied topically to remove unwanted hair.

Depression, respiratory   (i) Abnormally low rate and depth of breathing. (ii) Reduction in the amount of oxygen available to tissues (*see also*: Hypoxia).

Derivative   A substance formed from a primary compound by chemical reaction.

Dermal   Relating to the skin.

Dermatitis   Inflammation of the skin.

Dermatitis herpetiformis   Disease characterized by the irregular occurrence of groups of intensely irritating skin lesions, the sites of which eventually become pigmented.

Descaling agent   Substance used to remove deposits from kettles and other vessels.

Detergent   A chemical cleaning agent.

Diabetes mellitus   Disorder of glucose metabolism due to insulin deficiency.

Dialysis   The separation of substances by diffusion through a semipermeable membrane.

Dialysis, peritoneal   Procedure whereby blood is purified by dialysis against fluid infused into the peritoneal cavity and subsequently removed. The aim is to remove unwanted compounds of low relative molecular mass from the circulation.

Diluent   A fluid used in dilution.

Diplopia   Double vision.

Discriminating power   The ability of a system to distinguish between a number of possibilities.

Disinhibition   Removal of restraints on behaviour.

Disorientation   Confused as to direction.

Disseminated intravascular coagulation   Blood clotting throughout the systemic circulation, but associated with abnormal bleeding.

Diuresis   Increased production of urine.

Diuresis, forced   Abnormally enhanced urine production, for example following administration of intravenous fluids or diuretics.

Diuretic   An agent that increases urine production.

Drug   A substance that, when administered to an organism or a system derived from an organism, may modify one or more of its functions.

Drug, controlled   A drug whose use is regulated by law.

Dysphagia   Difficulty in swallowing.

Dyspnoea   Difficult or laboured breathing.

Dystonic reaction   A consequence of an alteration in the tone of a tissue.

Elimination half-life   *See* Plasma half-life.

Embalm   To preserve a body after death.

Emesis   Vomiting.

Emetic   Substance causing emesis.

Encephalopathy   Degenerative brain disease.

Enteral   Within the intestine; usually used to refer to oral administration of an agent.

Enterohepatic recirculation   A cycle in which substances excreted in bile are reabsorbed from the intestine.

Epigastric   Concerned with the part of the abdomen extending from the sternum to the umbilicus (epigastrum).

Erythrocyte   Red blood cell.

Euphoria   An exaggerated feeling of well-being.

Euthanasia   The bringing about of a gentle and easy death in the case of incurable and painful disease.

Fibrillation, ventricular   Serious loss of coordination in the contraction of the muscle fibres of the ventricles of the heart, leading to cessation of blood flow from the heart.

Fibrosis   The development of abnormal connective tissue, usually as a response to injury.

First-pass metabolism   The fraction of an oral dose metabolized in the liver or gut wall before reaching the systemic circulation.

Fumigant   A vapour used to kill pests.

Fungicide   A pesticide used to kill fungi or check the growth of spores.

Gag reflex   Automatic response which normally prevents inhalation of vomit by closing the epiglottis, the cartilaginous flap over the trachea.

Gastric   Relating to the stomach.

Gastritis   Inflammation of the stomach.

Gastroenteritis   Inflammation of the lining of the stomach and intestine.

Gastrointestinal   Relating to the stomach and intestine.

Genitourinary   Relating to the genitalia and the urinary system.

Granulocyte   A type of white blood cell.

Haematemesis   Vomiting of blood.

Haematocrit   Erythrocyte volume fraction; the ratio by volume of the blood cells to plasma.

Haematoma   Swelling composed of blood.

Haematuria   Blood in the urine.

Haemodialysis   Procedure whereby blood is dialysed against a large volume of isotonic fluid outside the body and then returned to the systemic circulation. Used to remove unwanted compounds of low relative molecular mass from the circulation.

Haemoglobin   An iron-containing pigment found in erythrocytes, which binds oxygen for transport within the bloodstream.

Haemolysis   Rupture of erythrocytes leading to the appearance of free haemoglobin in the plasma.

Haemoperfusion   Procedure whereby blood is passed through a column of adsorbent material outside the body and then returned to the systemic circulation. Used to remove unwanted components of low relative molecular mass from the circulation.

Haemorrhage   Bleeding.

Haemostasis   Stoppage of bleeding.

Halide   A compound consisting of halogen ions together with metallic or organic counter-ions.

Hallucination   An imagined occurrence, either visual or auditory.

Hallucinogen   A substance causing a hallucination.

Halogen   A member of the series of elements consisting, for practical purposes, of fluorine, chlorine, bromine and iodine.

Headspace   The space above a solid or liquid in a container.

Hepatic   Relating to the liver.

Hepatitis   Inflammation of the liver.

Hepatorenal   Relating to the liver and kidneys.

Hepatotoxic   Harmful to the liver.

Herbicide   A pesticide used to control or kill plants or plant seeds.

Histamine   An amine present in many tissues, release of which can cause dilatation of the capillary blood vessels, flushing and other effects.

Hydrolysis   Decomposition caused by or involving water.

Hydrophilic   Readily soluble in water.

Hydrophobic   Not readily soluble in water.

Hyperactive   Abnormally active.

Hyperbilirubinaemia   An excess of bilirubin in the blood.

Hypercalcaemia   Abnormally high blood calcium concentration.

Hyperglycaemia   Abnormally high blood sugar (glucose) concentration.

Hyperkalaemia   Abnormally high blood potassium concentration.

Hypernatraemia   Abnormally high blood sodium concentration.

Hyperpnoea   Abnormally rapid and deep breathing (*see also*: Hyperventilation, Tachypnoea).

Hyperpyrexia   Abnormally high body temperature.

Hyperreflexia   Abnormally exaggerated reflexes.

Hypersalivation   Excessive production of saliva.

Hypertension   Abnormally high blood pressure.

Hyperthermia   Dangerously high body temperature.

Hyperventilation   Increased rate and depth of respiration (*see also* Hyperpnoea).

Hypnotic   Capable of inducing sleep.

Hypocalcaemia   Abnormally low blood calcium concentration.

Hypoglycaemia   Abnormally low blood sugar (glucose) concentration.

Hypokalaemia   Abnormally low blood potassium concentration.

Hypophosphataemia   Abnormally low blood phosphate concentration.

Hypostatic   Caused by the combined effects of gravity and poor circulation of the blood.

Hypotension   Abnormally low blood pressure.

Hypothermia   Abnormally low body temperature.

Hypotonia   Abnormally low muscle tone.

Hypoxia   Reduction of oxygen in an animal body below physiological requirements (*see also*: Anoxia; Depression, respiratory).

Iatrogenic   Induced in a patient by the comments or treatment of a physician. Used especially in connection with inappropriate drug treatment.

Incontinence   Lack of voluntary control over the discharge of urine or faeces.

Inebriation   Excitement or elation induced by alcohol or other drugs.

Inflammation   Soreness and pain in joints or other parts of the body.

Ingestion   Taking of substances into the body by mouth.

Inotrope   An agent that increases or decreases the contractility of the heart muscle.

Insecticide   A pesticide used to control or kill insects.

Inspiration   The act of breathing in.

Intoxication   (i) Poisoning. (ii) Inebriation.

Ischaemia   Deficiency of blood supply to a part of the body.

Isobestic point   Wavelength at which the specific absorbances of two interconvertible materials are the same, regardless of the equilibrium position of the reaction between them.

Isotonic   Having the same osmolality.

Jaundice   Disease characterized by the deposition of yellow bile pigments in, for example, the eyes and skin.

Ketoacidosis   Metabolic acidosis due to the production of excessive amounts of ketones such as acetone.

Ketonuria   The presence of excessive amounts of ketones, such as acetone, in urine, often indicating a disorder of glucose metabolism, such as diabetes mellitus, but sometimes due simply to starvation.

Lacrimation   The secretion of tears.

Leishmaniasis   Disease caused by infection with a protozoon transmitted to humans by sandflies.

Leukocyte   White blood cell.

Leukocyte count   Concentration of white blood cells in a sample of blood.

Limit of detection   The smallest amount of a substance that can be revealed by a test carried out in a prescribed manner.

Lipaemia   The presence of abnormal amounts of fats in the blood.

Lipophilic   Readily soluble in fats and organic solvents.

Lipophobic   Not readily soluble in fats and organic solvents.

Maintenance therapy   Planned, long-term drug therapy; for example, treatment of opiate dependence with methadone.

Malaise   Feeling of discomfort or sickness.

Mania   Mental illness characterized by elation, excessively rapid speech and violent, destructive actions.

MAOI   *See* Monoamine oxidase inhibitor.

Metabolism   Chemical reactions occurring in organisms or in systems derived from organisms, whereby the function of nutrition is effected.

Metabolite   A substance produced by metabolism.

Methaemoglobin   Oxidized haemoglobin.

Methaemoglobinaemia   The presence of abnormal amounts of oxidized haemoglobin in the blood.

Miosis   Contraction of the pupil of the eye (cf. Mydriasis).

Mixer, rotary   A device for mixing solutions or suspensions by means of a gentle rotating motion. Used for solvent extraction or other procedures requiring mixing of relatively large quantities of material (cf. Vortex-mixer).

Monoamine oxidase inhibitor An antidepressant that acts by inhibiting the metabolism of amines acting as neurotransmitters in the brain.

Mydriasis Extreme dilatation of the pupil of the eye.

Myocardial Relating to the myocardium, the muscle of the heart.

Myoclonus A sudden shock-like muscular contraction which may involve one or more muscles or a few fibres of a muscle.

Myoglobin A protein related to haemoglobin, found in muscle.

Myoglobinuria The presence of myoglobin in the urine.

Narcotic An agent that produces insensibility or stupor (narcosis).

Nausea A feeling of need to vomit.

Necrosis Cell death due to anoxia or local toxic or microbiological action. Used particularly to describe cell death at a focal point in a multicellular organism.

Neonatal Newly born.

Nephrotoxic Harmful to the kidney.

Neuroleptic A drug that produces analgesia, sedation and tranquillization; used in the treatment of psychosis.

Neuropathy, peripheral Disease characterized by disintegration or destruction of the specialized tissues of the peripheral nervous system.

Neuropsychiatric Relating to the nervous system and mental processes.

Neurotoxic Harmful to nerve tissue.

Neurotransmitter Compound, e.g. acetylcholine, responsible for transmission of nerve impulses at synapses.

Nystagmus Constant, involuntary, jerky eye movement.

Ocular Relating to the eye.

Oedema Pathological accumulation of fluid in tissue spaces.

Oliguria Production of a diminished amount of urine (cf. Anuria, Polyuria).

Ophthalmic Relating to the eye.

Opiate   A pharmacologically active agent, such as morphine, derived from opium.

Opioid   An agent that has agonist activity at specific receptors in the brain.

Opium   The dried juice of the poppy *Papaver somniferum*.

Opisthotonos   Extreme arching backwards of the spine and neck as a result of muscle spasm.

Osmolality   The osmotic strength of a solution.

Osmotic   Relating to osmosis.

Osteomalacia   Softening of bones as a result of loss of calcium salts.

Palpitations   Abnormal awareness of the heartbeat.

Pancreatitis   Inflammation of the pancreas.

Papilloedema   Oedema of the optic nerve-head.

Paraesthesia   Numbness and tingling.

Paralysis   Loss of power in any part of the body.

Paralytic ileus   Distension of the intestine due to paralysis of the muscle of the intestinal wall.

Parenteral   By some means other than through the intestinal canal. Usually used to refer to intramuscular, intraperitoneal or intravenous administration of a substance.

Parkinsonism   A syndrome characterized by muscle rigidity, hand tremor, mask-like facial expression and other features.

Parotid gland   Salivary gland near to the ear.

Perinatal   In humans, relating to the period between the twenty-second week of pregnancy and the first week after birth.

Pesticide   Substance used to kill or control any pest, including animals, plants, fungi, or other organisms in agricultural, industrial and domestic situations.

Petechiae   Small red or purple spots caused by accumulation of blood beneath the skin.

Pharmacokinetics   The action of drugs in the body over a period of time, including the processes of absorption, distribution, metabolism and elimination.

Phenylketonuria   Inherited disorder of phenylalanine metabolism characterized by the appearance of phenylpyruvic acid in the urine.

Phosphorylation, oxidative   Electron transport process whereby energy released by oxidation of products from the tricarboxylic acid cycle in mitochondria is stored initially as adenosine triphosphate.

Pin-point pupils   Extreme contraction of the pupils of the eyes (*see also* Miosis).

Pipette, automatic   Device used to dispense repeatedly known volumes of a fluid.

Pipette, positive-displacement   Device with a washable tip, used to take up and dispense known volumes of a fluid, and in which the plunger is in contact with the fluid. Used to dispense viscous solutions such as whole blood.

Pipette, semi-automatic   Device, often with disposable tips, used to take up and dispense known volumes of aqueous fluids such as plasma or serum. Reliable only for fluids with a viscosity similar to that of water.

Plasma   The fluid portion ot circulating blood (cf. Serum).

Plasma half-life   The time taken for the plasma concentration of a substance to decrease by half.

Platelet count   The concentration of platelets in a sample of blood.

Pneumonitis   Inflammation of the lung.

Poison   A chemical that may harm or kill an organism.

Polyuria   Production of an excessive amount of urine (cf. Anuria, Oliguria).

Prophylaxis   Treatment intended to prevent the occurrence of disease.

Protective agent   Substance that can prevent the manifestations of toxicity of an agent on an organism (cf. Antidote).

Protein binding   Non-covalent adherence of drugs and other agents to protein. In plasma, acidic compounds normally bind to albumin and bases may also bind to α_1-acid glycoprotein.

Proteinaemia   The presence of excessive amounts of protein in blood.

Prothrombin time   A measure of the time taken for blood to clot *in vitro*. Often reported as a ratio to a control (normal) value.

Psychoactive   Affecting the brain and influencing behaviour; psychotropic.

Psychosis   A serious mental disorder characterized by confusion, delusions, and hallucinations.

Psychotropic   Affecting the brain and influencing behaviour; psychoactive.

Pulmonary   Relating to the lungs.

Putrefaction   Process of decomposition occurring in dead tissue.

Pyrexia   Raised body temperature; fever.

Reconstitute   Redissolve a solute after removal of a solvent.

Relative density   The ratio of the density of a material to the density of a reference material, usually water.

Renal   Relating to the kidneys.

Repellent   A substance used to drive away pests, such as insects.

Rhabdomyolysis   Muscle breakdown leading to the appearance of myoglobin in blood and urine.

Rodenticide   Pesticide used to control or kill rats or other rodents.

Rubefacient   Causing reddening of the skin.

Salicylism   Chronic poisoning caused by excessive use of salicylates. Characterized by respiratory alkalosis followed by metabolic acidosis.

Scene residue   Material found at the scene of a poisoning incident.

Schistosomiasis   Infection with trematode parasitic flukes of the genus *Schistosoma*.

Schizophrenia   A form of psychosis in which there are fundamental distortions of thinking and perception. Delusions and hallucinations are common clinical features.

Screening   (i) In clinical toxicology, a search for unknown poisons by chemical analysis of biological or other specimens (drug screen, poisons screen). (ii) In experimental toxicology, a search for possible toxicity of a substance in normal use (safety screen).

Sedative   An agent that quiets nervous excitement; used to treat agitation.

Sensitivity   An indication of the minimum quantity of a substance that can be detected and identified by a test.

Sequelae   Consequences of disease or injury.

Sequestrant   A substance that removes an ion or renders it ineffective (*see also*: Chelate).

Serum   (i) The clear, usually watery, fluid that moistens the surface of internal membranes. (ii) The watery portion of blood which remains after blood clots (cf. Plasma).

Shock   The general metabolic and other consequences of severe injury, characterized by low body temperature, low blood pressure, rapid pulse, pale, cold, moist skin and, often, vomiting, restlessness and anxiety.

Sign   Objective evidence of disease or of an effect induced by a poison, perceptible to an examining physician (cf. Symptom).

Spike   In analytical chemistry, to add a known amount of a pure compound to a blank specimen to act as a positive control.

Spray reagent   *See* Visualization reagent.

Stasis   Stoppage.

Stellate ganglion block   Procedure in which local anaesthesia is induced in the branch of the inferior cervical ganglion concerned with vision.

Stimulant   An agent that increases activity, for example in the central nervous system.

Stomatitis   Inflammation of the mucous membrane of the mouth.

Stupor   Lethargy; torpor; unconsciousness.

Subclinical   Describes changes resulting from disease or intoxication that do not produce clinically recognizable symptoms.

Sublingual   Beneath the tongue.

Submaxillary gland   Salivary gland situated beneath the lower jaw.

Supernatant   An upper layer of liquid.

Sympathomimetic   A drug that mimics the action of endogenous neurotransmitters in the sympathetic nervous system.

Symptom   Subjective evidence of disease or intoxication as perceived by the patient (cf. Sign).

Synapse   Area of contact between two nerve cells.

Syncope   Loss of consciousness caused by a sudden fall of blood pressure in the brain.

Synergist   A substance that increases the effect of another.

Systemic   Affecting the body as a whole.

Tachyarrhythmia   An arrhythmia associated with an excessively rapid heart-beat.

Tachycardia   Excessively rapid heartbeat.

Tachypnoea   Unduly rapid breathing (cf. Hyperpnoea).

Tetany   Heightened excitability of the motor nerves with painful muscle cramps.

Thrombocytopenia   Abnormally low number of platelets in the blood.

Tinnitus   A continual noise in the ears, such as ringing, buzzing, roaring or clicking.

Tolerance   (i) The ability of an organism to experience exposure to potentially harmful amounts of a poison without showing evidence of toxicity. (ii) An adaptive state whereby the pharmacological effects of the same dose of a substance become diminished as a result of repeated exposure.

Toxin   A poison of natural origin.

Toxic   Able to cause injury to living organisms as a result of chemical interaction within the organism.

Toxicity   Any harmful effect of a chemical on an organism.

Toxicology   The study of the actual or potential danger to organisms presented by the harmful effects of chemicals.

Tranquillizer   A drug used to treat anxiety.

Tremor   Shaking or quivering, especially in the hands.

Tricarboxylic acid cycle   Citric acid cycle, Krebs cycle: intermediary metabolic sequence whereby energy from fats and sugars is made available for oxidative phosphorylation, among other functions.

Tricyclic antidepressant   Drug, such as amitriptyline, characterized by the presence of three conjugated aromatic rings and used to treat depression.

Tuberculosis   A disease caused by *Mycobacterium tuberculosis*, characterized by the development of nodules (tubercules) in affected tissues, for example the lung.

Ulcer, peptic   An ulcer of the stomach or duodenum.

Ulceration   Formation of open sores.

Uraemia   The clinical state arising from kidney failure; literally, excess urea in the blood.

Urinary retention   Abnormal retention of urine in the bladder.

Urticaria   An acute or chronic dermatitis characterized by the presence of white, red or pink spots on the skin accompanied by itching, stinging or burning sensations.

Vasodilatation   Dilatation (expansion) of a blood vessel leading to increased flow of blood through the vessel.

Vehicle   A substance with which a drug or other substance is mixed for administration or application.

Vertigo   A sensation of dizziness, leading to loss of balance.

Viscosity   (of a fluid) Resistance to flow.

Visualization reagent   A substance or solution used to reveal the presence of other substances on thin-layer chromatograms, for example.

Volume of distribution   Theoretical relationship, useful as an indicator of tissue distribution, between the amount of a drug or other compound in the body (d mg) and the concentration of the compound measured in whole blood or in plasma/serum (c mg/l):

Volume of distribution $= d/c$ litres.

Water-soluble compounds such as phenazone (see section 6.39) have a volume of distribution comparable to the volume of water in the body, while lipophilic compounds such as digoxin (see section 6.41) have a volume of distribution many times greater.

Relative volume of distribution is volume of distribution divided by body weight.

Vortex-mixer   A device for mixing solutions or suspensions by means of a whirling motion which creates a cavity in the centre of the mixture. Used for solvent extraction and other procedures requiring efficient mixing of relatively small quantities of material (up to about 10 ml total volume) (cf. Mixer, rotary).

Withdrawal, drug   The act or consequences of reduction or cessation of drug administration in a dependent subject. The clinical features observed (commonly sweating, tremor, nausea, vomiting) are often reversible if drug use is recommenced (*see also* Delirium tremens).

Xenobiotic   Compound foreign to the metabolism of an organism.

List of reference compounds and reagents

The reference compounds and reagents required for the tests are listed here. A number are controlled drugs and special arrangements are necessary to obtain and store these items (see section 1.2). Where appropriate, the commonly encountered salts of basic drugs and some other compounds have been indicated. Compounds marked with an asterisk (*) are used both as reagents and reference compounds.

Reference compounds

Pharmaceuticals and metabolites

N-Acetylprocainamide (hydrochloride)
Acetylsalicylic acid
Amitriptyline (hydrochloride)
Amobarbital
Amfetamine (sulfate)
Atropine (sulfate)

Barbital (sodium)
Benzoylecgonine
Bisacodyl
Brucine (sulfate)

Caffeine
Carbamazepine
Chloroquine (phosphate)
Chlorpromazine (hydrochloride)
Clomethiazole (ethandisulfonate)
Clomipramine (hydrochloride)
Cocaine
Codeine (phosphate)
Cyclizine (hydrochloride)

Dantron
Dapsone
Desipramine (hydrochloride)
Dextropropoxyphene (hydrochloride)
Digoxin
Digitoxin
Dihydrocodeine (tartrate)

Diphenhydramine (hydrochloride)
Dosulepin (hydrochloride)
Doxepin (hydrochloride)

Emetine (hydrochloride)
Ephedrine (hydrochloride)
Ethchlorvynol

Flurazepam (hydrochloride)

Glutethimide
Glyceryl trinitrate (aqueous solution)

Haloperidol

Imipramine (hydrochloride)*
Isoniazid

Lidocaine (hydrochloride)
Lithium (carbonate)

Meprobamate
Methadone (hydrochloride)
Methaqualone
Metamfetamine (hydrochloride)
Methyprylon
Monoacetyldapsone
Morphine (sulfate)
Morphine-3-glucuronide

Nitrazepam
Nortriptyline (hydrochloride)

Orphenadrine (citrate)

Paracetamol
Pentazocine (hydrochloride)
Perphenazine
Pethidine (hydrochloride)
Phenazone
Phenobarbital
Phenolphthalein
Phenytoin
Pralidoxime (chloride)*
Procainamide (hydrochloride)
Propranolol (hydrochloride)

Quinidine (sulfate)
Quinine (sulfate)*

Rhein

Salicylic acid
Strychnine (hydrochloride)

Theophylline
Thioridazine (hydrochloride)
Trifluoperazine (hydrochloride)
Trimipramine (maleate)
Tolbutamide

Verapamil (hydrochloride)

Pesticides

Aldicarb
Aldrin

Bromophos
Bromoxynil

Carbaryl
Chloralose
Chlorpyrifos

2, 4-D
DNOC
2, 4-DP
Dicophane
Dimethoate
Dinoseb
Dioxathion
Diquat

Heptachlor

Ioxynil

Lindane

MCPA
MCPP
Methidathion
Methiocarb

Nicotine

Paraquat
Pentachlorophenol
2, 4, 5-T
2, 4, 5-TP

Reagents and solvents

Acetaldehyde
Acetamide
Acetic acid (glacial)
Acetic anhydride
Acetone
Acetylthiocholine iodide
Alcohol dehydrogenase (yeast, crystalline, see page 132)
Alizarin complexone
2-Aminoethanol
1-Aminonaphthalene
Ammonium acetate
Ammonium chloride
Ammonium hydroxide (concentrated, relative density 0.88)
Ammonium molybdate
Ammonium sulfamate
Ammonium sulfate
Ammonium thiocyanate
Ammonium vanadate (finely powdered)
iso-Amyl acetate
Arsenic trichloride

Barbituric acid (malonylurea, 2,4,6-trihydroxypyrimidine)
Basic magenta (fuchsine, CI 42510)
2,2'-Bipyridyl (2,2'-dipyridyl)
Boric acid*
Bromine
Butanone (methyl ethyl ketone)
n-Butyl acetate

Calcium chloride
Calcium hydroxide
Calcium hypochlorite (powdered)
Carbon monoxide* (or carbon monoxide/nitrogen, see page 97)
Carminic acid
Cerous nitrate
Charcoal, activated (Norit A)
Chloramine T (*N*-chloro-4-toluenesulfonamide, sodium salt; see note, page 119)
Chloroauric acid (gold chloride, $HAuCl_4 \cdot xH_2O$)
Chloroform
Chromotropic acid (2,5-dihydroxynaphthalene-2,7-disulfonic acid)
Citric acid
Copper foil, mesh or wire*
o-Cresol (2-methylphenol)
Copper (II) sulfate
Cyclohexane

Diethyl ether
p-Dimethylaminobenzaldehyde (4-dimethylaminobenzaldehyde)
p-Dimethylaminocinnamaldehyde (4-dimethylaminocinnamaldehyde)

o-Dinitrobenzene (1,2-dinitrobenzene)
Dinitrophenol
Diphenylamine
Diphenylamine sulfate
Diphenylcarbazide
Disodium hydrogen orthophosphate
Disodium tetraborate
5,5'-Dithiobis(2-nitrobenzoic acid) (Ellman's reagent)
Dithiooxamide
Dithizone (diphenylthiocarbazone)

Ethanol*
Ethyl acetate

Ferric ammonium sulfate*
Ferric chloride
Ferric nitrate (nonahydrate)
Ferrous sulfate
Fluorescein
1-Fluoro-2,4-dinitrobenzene
Folin-Ciocalteau reagent (see page 202)
Formaldehyde* (see page 220)
Formic acid*
Furfuraldehyde

Glycine

n-Hexane
Hippuric acid*
Hydrochloric acid (concentrated, relative density 1.18)
Hydrogen peroxide*

Iodine
Isopropyl acetone

Ketodase (β-glucuronidase 5000 units/ml)

Lead acetate*
Lithium sulfate

Magnesium (powder)
Manganous sulfate
Mercuric chloride*
Mercurous nitrate
Metaphosphoric acid
Methanol*
2-Methoxyethanol (ethylene glycol monomethyl ether)
Methyl *iso*-butyl ketone (isopropylacetone)
Methyl tertiary-butyl ether

N-(1-Naphthyl)ethylenediamine hydrochloride
Nicotinamide adenine dinucleotide (see page 132)
Nitric acid (concentrated, relative density 1.42)
p-Nitrobenzaldehyde (4-nitrobenzaldehyde)
4-(p-Nitrobenzyl)pyridine (4-(4-nitrobenzyl)pyridine)

Orthophosphoric acid (o-phosphoric acid, H_3PO_4) (850 g/kg)
Oxalyldihydrazide (oxalylhydrazide)
Oxalic acid*

Paraffin wax
Perchloric acid (700 g/kg)
Petroleum ether (40–60 °C boiling fraction)
Phenol*
Phosphorous acid (metaphosphoric acid, H_3PO_3)
Platinic chloride (platinum (IV) chloride)
Potassium cyanide*
Potassium dichromate
Potassium ferricyanide (hexacyanoferrate (III))
Potassium ferrocyanide (hexacyanoferrate (II))
Potassium iodide
Potassium nitrite
Potassium permanganate
Potassium sodium tartrate tetrahydrate (Rochelle salt)
Potassium thiocyanate*
Propan-2-ol*
Pyridine

Salicylaldehyde (2-hydroxybenzaldehyde)
Semicarbazide hydrochloride (N-aminourea hydrochloride, see page 132)
Silica (precipitated)
Silver dithiocarbamate
Silver nitrate
Sodium acetate, anhydrous
Sodium acetate dihydrate
Sodium azide
Sodium bicarbonate
Sodium bisulfite
Sodium bitartrate
Sodium bromide*
Sodium carbonate
Sodium chlorate*
Sodium chloride
Sodium dihydrogen orthophosphate
Sodium dithionite (N.B. This compound must be stored in a desiccator)
Sodium hydrogen orthophosphate
Sodium hydroxide
Sodium hypochlorite*
Sodium fluoride*
Sodium iodate*
Sodium iodide*

Sodium molybdate
Sodium nitrate*
Sodium nitrite*
Sodium nitroprusside
Sodium periodate
Sodium pyrophosphate (tetra-sodium pyrophosphate decahydrate)
Sodium rhodizonate (rhodizonic acid, sodium salt)
Sodium sulfate (anhydrous)
Sodium sulfide*
Sodium sulfite*
Sodium tungstate
Stannous chloride
Starch (solid)
Sulfanilic acid
Sulfuric acid (concentrated, relative density 1.83)

Tartaric acid
Tergitol
Tetraethylenepentamine
Thallous sulfate*
Thiobarbituric acid (4,6-dihydroxy-2-mercaptopyrimidine)
Toluene
o-Toluidine (2-methylaniline)
Trichloroacetic acid*
Triethylamine
Tris(hydroxymethyl)aminomethane (free base)
Turmeric (the spice, see page 83)

Urea

m-Xylene (1,3-dimethylbenzene)

Zinc (granulated)
Zinc acetate
Zinc phosphide*

Conversion factors for mass and molar concentrations

The units given here are those normally used to report the results of measurements performed on fluids such as blood or urine.

Analyte	Mass/molar	Molar/mass
Acetylsalicylic acid	*see* salicylate ion	
Aluminium	$\mu g/l \times 0.0371 = \mu mol/l$	$\mu mol/l \times 27 = \mu g/l$
Amitriptyline	$\mu g/l \times 0.00361 = \mu mol/l$	$\mu mol/l \times 277 = \mu g/l$
Arsenic	$mg/l \times 13.3 = \mu mol/l$	$\mu mol/l \times 0.0749 = mg/l$
Barbital	$mg/l \times 5.43 = \mu mol/l$	$\mu mol/l \times 0.184 = mg/l$
Borate ion	$mg/l \times 17.0 = \mu mol/l$	$\mu mol/l \times 0.0588 = mg/l$
Bromide ion	$mg/l \times 12.52 = \mu mol/l$	$\mu mol/l \times 0.0799 = mg/l$
Bromoxynil	$mg/l \times 3.61 = \mu mol/l$	$\mu mol/l \times 0.277 = mg/l$
Cadmium	$\mu g/l \times 8.90 = nmol/l$	$nmol/l \times 0.112 = \mu g/l$
Carbamazepine	$mg/l \times 4.24 = \mu mol/l$	$\mu mol/l \times 0.236 = mg/l$
Chloroquine	$mg/l \times 3.13 = \mu mol/l$	$\mu mol/l \times 0.320 = mg/l$
Clomethiazole	$mg/l \times 6.17 = \mu mol/l$	$\mu mol/l \times 0.162 = mg/l$
Copper	$mg/l \times 15.7 = \mu mol/l$	$\mu mol/l \times 0.0636 = mg/l$
Cyanide	$mg/l \times 38.5 = \mu mol/l$	$\mu mol/l \times 0.026 = mg/l$
Dapsone	$mg/l \times 4.03 = \mu mol/l$	$\mu mol/l \times 0.248 = mg/l$
Diazepam	$mg/l \times 3.51 = \mu mol/l$	$\mu mol/l \times 0.285 = mg/l$
Digoxin	$\mu g/l \times 1.28 = nmol/l$	$nmol/l \times 0.781 = \mu g/l$
Dinoseb	$mg/l \times 4.17 = \mu mol/l$	$\mu mol/l \times 0.240 = mg/l$
DNOC	$mg/l \times 5.05 = \mu mol/l$	$\mu mol/l \times 0.198 = mg/l$
Ethanol	$g/l \times 21.7 = mmol/l$	$mmol/l \times 0.046 = g/l$
Ethylene glycol	$g/l \times 16.1 = mmol/l$	$mmol/l \times 0.062 = g/l$
Fluoride ion	$mg/l \times 52.6 = \mu mol/l$	$\mu mol/l \times 0.019 = mg/l$
Hippurate ion	$g/l \times 5.61 = mmol/l$	$mmol/l \times 0.178 = g/l$
Imipramine	$\mu g/l \times 0.00357 = \mu mol/l$	$\mu mol/l \times 280 = \mu g/l$
Ioxynil	$mg/l \times 2.696 = \mu mol/l$	$\mu mol/l \times 0.371 = mg/l$
Iron	$mg/l \times 17.9 = \mu mol/l$	$\mu mol/l \times 0.0559 = mg/l$
Isoniazid	$mg/l \times 7.29 = \mu mol/l$	$\mu mol/l \times 0.137 = mg/l$
Lead	$mg/l \times 4.83 = \mu mol/l$	$\mu mol/l \times 0.207 = mg/l$
Lidocaine	$mg/l \times 4.27 = \mu mol/l$	$\mu mol/l \times 0.234 = mg/l$
Lithium	$mg/l \times 0.144 = mmol/l$	$mmol/l \times 6.94 = mg/l$

Mercury	$\mu g/l \times 4.99 = nmol/l$	$nmol/l \times 0.201 = \mu g/l$
Methanol	$g/l \times 31.3 = mmol/l$	$mmol/l \times 0.032 = g/l$
Methaqualone	$mg/l \times 4.00 = \mu mol/l$	$\mu mol/l \times 0.250 = mg/l$
Morphine	$mg/l \times 3.51 = \mu mol/l$	$\mu mol/l \times 0.285 = mg/l$
Nitrite ion	$mg/l \times 21.7 = \mu mol/l$	$\mu mol/l \times 0.046 = mg/l$
Nortriptyline	$mg/l \times 3.80 = \mu mol/l$	$\mu mol/l \times 0.263 = mg/l$
Paracetamol	$mg/l \times 0.00661 = mmol/l$	$mmol/l \times 151 = mg/l$
Paraquat ion	$mg/l \times 5.37 = \mu mol/l$	$\mu mol/l \times 0.186 = mg/l$
Phenobarbital	$mg/l \times 4.31 = \mu mol/l$	$\mu mol/l \times 0.232 = mg/l$
Phenprocoumon	$mg/l \times 3.57 = \mu mol/l$	$\mu mol/l \times 0.280 = mg/l$
Phenytoin	$mg/l \times 3.96 = \mu mol/l$	$\mu mol/l \times 0.252 = mg/l$
Primidone	$mg/l \times 4.58 = \mu mol/l$	$\mu mol/l \times 0.218 = mg/l$
Propan-2-ol	$g/l \times 16.64 = mmol/l$	$mmol/l \times 0.060 = g/l$
Quinidine	$mg/l \times 3.08 = \mu mol/l$	$\mu mol/l \times 0.325 = mg/l$
Salicylate ion	$mg/l \times 0.00729 = mmol/l$	$mmol/l \times 137 = mg/l$
Sulfite ion	$mg/l \times 12.5 = \mu mol/l$	$\mu mol/l \times 0.080 = mg/l$
Thallium	$mg/l \times 4.89 = \mu mol/l$	$\mu mol/l \times 0.204 = mg/l$
Theophylline	$mg/l \times 5.55 = \mu mol/l$	$\mu mol/l \times 0.180 = mg/l$
Thiocyanate ion	$mg/l \times 17.2 = \mu mol/l$	$\mu mol/l \times 0.058 = mg/l$
Tolbutamide	$mg/l \times 3.70 = \mu mol/l$	$\mu mol/l \times 0.270 = mg/l$
Valproate ion	$mg/l \times 6.98 = \mu mol/l$	$\mu mol/l \times 0.143 = mg/l$
Warfarin	$mg/l \times 3.24 = \mu mol/l$	$\mu mol/l \times 0.308 = mg/l$
Zinc	$mg/l \times 15.3 = \mu mol/l$	$\mu mol/l \times 0.0654 = mg/l$

Index

Selected WHO publications of related interest

	Price (Sw. fr.)*
Manual of basic techniques for a health laboratory. 1980 (478 pages)	30.–
Laboratory biosafety manual, 2nd ed. 1993 (144 pages)	26.–
Biosafety guidelines for diagnostic and research laboratories working with HIV. WHO AIDS Series, No. 9, 1991 (32 pages)	8.–
Basic tests for pharmaceutical substances. 1986 (210 pages)	34.–
Basic tests for pharmaceutical dosage forms. 1991 (134 pages)	24.–
Management of poisoning. A handbook for health care personnel. J. Henry & H. Wiseman (in press)	
Guidelines for poison control centres (in press)	

Further information on these and other WHO publications can be obtained from Distribution and Sales, World Health Organization, 1211 Geneva 27, Switzerland.

*Prices in developing countries are 70% of those listed here.

www.ingramcontent.com/pod-product-compliance
Lightning Source LLC
Chambersburg PA
CBHW050900210326
41597CB00002B/32